Everything I Learned About Perimenopausal Migraines

Kirsty Campbell

for Kate
in case this is future you

for Ian
for always picking up the pieces

Ten years ago, I began suffering from perimenopausal migraines, at the age of 39. I went from having the occasional migraine attack to living with migraine 75% of the time. Over the past decade, I feel like I have tried everything to make the pain and other symptoms better - sometimes with success, sometimes not so much. I wanted to share what worked (and didn't) to try to help other perimenopausal migraine sufferers.

I am a therapist with ten years of experience and I also share some case studies of people I've supported through similar struggles. There are certainly many ways to navigate the perimenopause, and the challenge of hormonal migraines in particular.

There are some great migraine books out there written by medical professionals, but not as much from the perspective of the sufferer. I suspect this is because most sufferers are hunched over a toilet bowl, trying to shield their eyes from bright light. But, now that I am coming out the other end of the tunnel, my hope is that writing about my own experience might give you some comfort and perhaps some tips and tricks.

You can find me at www.kirsty-campbell.com

Table of Contents

Introduction 5
What is perimenopause? 7
What is a migraine? 9
And what is a perimenopausal migraine? 11
My personal experience with migraines 13
Case studies 40
Anita – finding ways to manage stress and guilt 40
Amanda – not letting it stop you (from travelling) 47
Nicole – managing nausea 52
Danielle – when it's trauma related 59
Summary 65
Ways I've managed perimenopausal migraines 67
Ways I've managed (good) 68
Painkillers 68
Triptans 72
Knowing about triggers 73
Friends 75
Migraine diary and pain scale 78
Sleep 84
Caffeine 87
Water 90
Food 92
Alcohol 95
Managing stress 98
Do things anyway 106
Dark glasses and eye shades 108
Ear plugs and noise cancelling headphones 109
Music 110
Ice packs 111
Thought games for the anxiety 111
Be prepared with your migraine first aid kit 113
Expect a migraine 115
Ways I've managed (bad) 117

Making no concessions for myself 117
Never cancelling work 119
Exercise 121
Overt violence 122
Dr Google 123
Stupid things people say about migraine 123
Hope for the future 127
What I have learned from perimenopausal migraines 128
Acknowledgements 132
About the author 133
References 134

Introduction

I have a very clear memory of "the period assembly". Perhaps you remember something similar. I was a newbie Year 7 at secondary school, and my form tutor announced that the assembly that morning was "just for the girls". The boys got to stay in their form rooms while us girls all trooped over to the hall in the rain. The reason for this, it turned out, was that the Deputy Head wanted to tell us a few things about starting our periods.

I hope that for most of the girls in the assembly room, none of what the Deputy Head had to say was news. My mum had done her duty and told me all about periods some time previously. But I know, from my experience since as both a teacher and a school counsellor, that some of them will have been hearing about what was going to happen to them soon for the first time. I think that's why they picked the Deputy Head to do this big talk. She was authoritative but also extremely kind and reassuring. She covered the main points: everything from what happens when you get your period to how to dispose of your sanitary towels. And although none of us planned to ever do this, she assured us that we could rock up to her office and ask for a tampon or a towel anytime if we were caught short.

I think it's great that my school did this. I hope that they still do it, and maybe talk to the boys about periods as well.

But what I've been thinking recently is, how would it be if, at some point in our late thirties, all of us women got called back into school so that an experienced woman could tell us about perimenopause? Imagine: we'd all somehow get an email at just the right time, and go about rearranging our busy professional and family calendars to take an hour off to go and get on the same page about what's about to happen to us as our periods come to an end.

We'd all jam back into that hall and some knowledgable Deputy Head figure would tell us about the likelihood that, sometime in the next few years, we'd start experiencing irregular periods, hot flushes, night sweats, bone deep fatigue, itchy skin, dry vaginas, sore boobs, mood swings, a loss of libido, actual murderous rage, heart palpitations, migraines, brain fog, insomnia, trouble concentrating, joint aches, muscle aches, bladder problems, weight gain, sprouting quite an impressive beard and matching moustache...and as the panic swept palpably through the packed hall, one brave soul would raise her hand and ask "OK, and how long will these symptoms last?" And the Deputy Head would say "Well, could be about ten years." There would be collective screech of TEN YEARS! and some much ruder words besides, from the women, many of whom would now be pale and sobbing.

Yeah, OK, I can see why no one does that assembly.

But the fact remains that education around perimenopause and menopause is very patchy. If you do all your research (and you can still manage that with your brain fog – well done you) then you're probably quite well self-informed. There have been some excellent documentaries, podcasts and social media accounts popping up over the past few years, too. We no longer have to refer to it in hushed tones as *the change* like our mothers and grandmothers did. However, we've got a long way to go. Women as elderly as their late forties are still being told by doctors that they're too young for their symptoms to be menopause related. They seem to have missed the basic stats: the average age for a woman to go through menopause is 51. The perimenopause lasts somewhere around four to ten years leading up to that point. It's an easy bit of maths.

My name is Kirsty, I'm 49 years old, and my particular peri struggle has been migraines. I have had perimenopausal migraines since I was 39. Over the past decade, I have tried all kinds of things to prevent and treat these migraines. I feel like I have accidentally become quite experienced in this area. I feel very lucky that I haven't had many of the catalogue of other perimenopausal symptoms that some women suffer from. But if perimenopausal migraines are your struggle too, I want to share with you the bits and pieces I've managed to pick up along the way. Everyone's pain is different, and your experience will not be exactly the same as mine, but if I save anyone from feeling like they're doing this whole thing from scratch, then that would make me very happy.

What is perimenopause?

The perimenopause is the span of time between which a woman first notices symptoms relating to her periods ending and the day on which she can say she hasn't had a period for one whole year. The perimenopause can last anywhere between a few months to over a decade, with the average time being around 4 years. It can affect a woman severely for the whole of that span of time, or just pop up intermittently, or anything in between. Some women even claim to experience no difficulties at all, but we don't talk about those lucky bitches.

Once a woman has not had a period for a whole year, she is considered to have gone through menopause, and be post-menopausal. So although we often talk about "the menopause" as this huge change, it really only lasts one day. I am assuming that is going to be a great day for me, for reasons you will soon come to understand, with streamers, balloons, party poppers and a large cake. I think it's the perimenopause, lasting so much longer and with such an array of symptoms, that is the real challenge. My post-menopausal friends tell me it is a new and bright world out the other side. Some people call it a "second spring" or a "new lease of life", which definitely sounds great. But it seems to me that there is something of a stormy winter to get through before it's time to start skipping through the tulips living your best wise woman life.

During perimenopause, not only are our periods winding down to a close, but several hormonal changes are occurring. The main one is that oestrogen levels fall as our ovaries stop working to produce eggs, and we come to the end of our fertile years. Our progesterone levels decrease too, since progesterone is no longer needed to prepare our bodies for and sustain pregnancy. It is also one of the biggest changes our bodies go through and what we know about change is that it isn't particularly easy.

It is a natural process, that all human females share, as well as some (not many) animals, including toothed whales and chimpanzees. Just because it is natural doesn't mean we have to go through it without help, though. The reason most animals don't go through a menopause is because it's been naturally selected out of most species – it's not efficient for them to keep females around who can't reproduce. Or, maybe, animals in their special wisdom researched perimenopause and said "fuck that shit – let's die instead." Either way, humans have opted to keep their wise older women around, which means we've got to work out this perimeno stuff.

Something that can be difficult to cope with is not only falling levels of hormones but fluctuating ones. Overall, our oestrogen and progesterone are going to take a nosedive, being present in much lower levels once we reach menopause than they were before the perimenopause started. However, during the perimenopause, levels of oestrogen and progesterone may temporarily surge as well as plunge, providing the least fun rollercoaster ever for our bodies and minds.

Oestrogen levels going through the roof can lead to mood swings, erratic periods, headaches and tiredness, while plummeting levels cause hot flushes, weight gain, erratic periods and anxiety. Surges in progesterone can cause breast tenderness, emotional highs and lows, water retention, weight gain and tiredness. Dips in progesterone can cause heavy, longer periods, sleeping problems, PMS, increases in anxiety and depression and also...migraines.

And yes, some of these symptoms look very similar, proving that having too much can be as hard as having too little – our bodies are like Goldilocks, wanting the levels to be "just right". Which is exactly what they hardly ever are during perimenopause.

It can really help to understand what is going on and why you feel alright one week and are plagued by a host of debilitating symptoms the next. But I feel like that's the first step. After that, I promise you, there are some treatment options. I know about all the ones for perimenopausal migraines and I'm going to talk in a lot of detail about them in this book. But please know that there is a lot of specific help out there for the myriad other symptoms of perimenopause too, so don't suffer alone or think you just have to be positive about it.

What is a migraine?

A migraine is different from a headache. A headache will typically be felt in your forehead as a constant pain and will usually resolve with paracetamol or sleep. By contrast, a migraine is typically on one side of your forehead or the other, is experienced as a pulsating or throbbing pain and often does not get better with simple painkillers or sleep. It may last several days and is often accompanied by nausea, sensitivity to light and/or sound and cognitive impairment. Migraine is a neurological disease that is not well understood and treatment can still be quite hit and miss.

Along with head pain, nausea, sensitivity to light/sound and brain fog, there are a lot of less obvious symptoms that can come with migraine. Gastrointestinal disturbance is common, as is insomnia, confusion, vertigo, needing to pee a lot, clumsiness and muscle stiffness. It's also not uncommon to experience irritability, low mood, depression, anxiety and even suicide ideation. The frequency of these additional symptoms tends to increase with the frequency and severity of the migraines.

Severe migraine attacks are classed by the World Health Organisation as among the most disabling illnesses to experience[i], on a par with dementia and psychosis.

Around 25-30% of migraine sufferers experience Migraine with Aura (MA) where the migraine pain is proceeded by visual disturbances. However, 70-75% (like me), experience Migraine without Aura (MO) where it's all about the pain and nausea.

Migraines affect around 15% of the population, with women affected four times as often as men. This is thought to be because oestrogen, one of the main female sex hormones, controls chemicals in our brains that are responsible for how we feel pain[ii]. In particular, oestrogen seems to impact how a pain molecule snappily named the calcitonin gene-related peptide (CGRP) functions. CGRP is thought to have a big role in migraine[iii]. Men, on the other hand, benefit from the slightly pain-protecting role that their main sex hormone, testosterone, has on pain signals. We women have testosterone in our systems, too, but at much lower levels.

Migraine is very heritable, with 90% of sufferers having at least one relative who is also a sufferer[iv]. So if your mother or grandmother suffered with migraines during her perimenopause, it may be that you will too.

A migraine attack typically lasts between 4 hours and 3 days, though my personal best is 17 days. For those suffers who experience MA, aura symptoms may be present for as much as a day or two before the migraine pain arrives. And for almost all sufferers, there is a "postdrome", or migraine hangover, where the pain has subsided but you feel exhausted.

If you experience migraines for more than 15 days in the month (oh, I've been there) then you have chronic migraine. It's not especially important to achieve that diagnosis to be honest, since the treatment is the same as for any other frequency of migraine, but it is definitely useful to talk to a doctor about it if you are at that stage and you haven't spoken to one already. And if any individual migraine attack lasts longer than 72 hours, then you are in Status Migrainosos. It's important to seek medical attention if your attack lasts this long in order to rule out some potential other causes but, assuming it is a migraine that's lasting more than three days, your body might need some assistance (a) coping with the lack of sleep, food and fluids and (b) getting some pain relief. I've been in Status Migrainosos hundreds of times and to be honest I didn't know what it was until I did the research for this book. I'm not suggesting you rock up at A&E every time your migraine goes over the 72 hour mark. Frankly, I'd have been subletting a cubicle from my local A&E if that were necessary. But the first time it happens, get it checked out to make sure it *is* migraine and then to get some advice. Once you know what you're doing with your migraine treatment, you will be able to start the drill yourself, and manage with support. But in the early days, it can be really scary, and you shouldn't hesitate to seek professional help.

The frequency of migraines varies a lot by individual, but the average frequency is three per month[v]. Some people will only have one or two per year and others will have more than one a week. I tend to think of mine in terms of how much time they take up, since attack frequency and duration can vary. I look at how many "migraine days" I've had per month versus how many days migraine-free. I think this helps when trying to look at the impact on your quality of life: after all, three migraines per month that last 4 hours each are going to feel different from three migraines per month that last 3 days each.

And what is a perimenopausal migraine?

If someone is a migraine sufferer before perimenopause, they are at higher risk of having more migraine attacks during perimenopause. This is because one of the triggers for migraine is hormonal changes, and hormones change a lot during the perimenopause. In particular, if you've suffered from PMS as well as migraines during your menstruating years, you may be more vulnerable to these changes in your hormones, and more likely to experience a worsening of migraines during perimenopause[vi].

As women you'd think we'd be used to our hormones changing. After all, that's what they've been doing every month, since shortly after we had that assembly in Year 7. Most of us have had some experience with period pain and PMS as a result of those monthly hormonal shifts. I don't want to diminish any of that, because for some of us that's bad enough (more on which, later). However, come perimenopause, those same hormones sort of rip up the rule book and instead of doing roughly the same dips and peaks at roughly the same time each month, they start doing whatever the fuck they like. They kind of go punk rock and experiment with dizzying peaks, deep old troughs and just generally trashing the place. Hence all those symptoms I listed can very much come and go unpredictably. As can the kind migraine you get during perimenopause.

Perimenopausal migraines differ from regular migraines in some quite depressing ways. It's all bad news, I'm afraid. Perimenopausal migraines tend to be more frequent, last longer and are more intense than regular migraines. In addition, they are harder to treat. This is because of the unpredictable nature of hormone fluctuations, though womens health generally is underfunded and less well understood[vii].

They are closely related to menstrual migraines, which are also worse than regular migraines in severity, duration, frequency and are less responsive to treatment[viii].

The only good news about perimenopausal migraines is that they are likely to either get a lot better or disappear completely some time after menopause[ix]. So, while they may be among the worst and most frequent migraines you can have, they are at least probably temporary. Although, by "temporary" I do mean somewhere in the region of a decade, depending on how long you're in perimenopause for and how long the migraines take to resolve after you've gone through the menopause.

My personal experience with migraines

I started my periods when I was 13 and, shortly after, had my first migraine. I had a very similar period experience to my mum (heavy, long lasting, painful periods) so she had already been through this and recognised the sharp pain that was pulsing behind my eyebrow. Thankfully, I only got a really bad migraine about once a year. I felt grateful for that, having tasted how miserable they were. Years later, I did get a lot more of them during pregnancy, but I was reassured that they would resolve within a few weeks, and they did.

Then, sometime in that year when I turned 40, I started getting a lot more migraines. I didn't keep records back then (oh how green I was! Nowadays I have stats and charts and graphs and you name it) but I think they were coming as regularly as once a month, but not in any particular pattern. Previously, they had always been tied to either the start or end of my period. Now, they just came whenever. And they might last a day, or three days – they really kept me guessing. I felt wiped out by them, especially when sometimes I'd only just got over one and the next one would start niggling away at my temple.

By the time I was 43, I was living with migraine 75% of the time. I realised I didn't know pain, or exhaustion, or cognitive impairment, until I hit this phase. My life was 75% migraine and 25% trying to recover from migraine. I did have a good GP, and we tried a lot of things (full details coming, read on) and sometimes it settled to a balance of 50% migraine, 50% migraine-free. But that was as good as it got for about five years.

My mum had told me that she got migraines during perimenopause too. "Not as many or as badly as you get them," she said, "but they did go away after menopause." I can't tell you how I hung onto that sentence. I had faith that, as horrible as this was, it was not going to last forever.

And it is easing up significantly. At 49, I am having two or three attacks a month. Sometimes they're much briefer than they used to be, sometimes not (my hormones are still a bit punk rock), but these days I'm migraining about 15-25% of the time. It's definitely going in a hopeful direction.

But that doesn't cancel out the fact that during these 10 years I have been compromised as a partner, a mum and a friend. While I've been having migraines, my husband has done an awful lot of my share of the chores. And my daughter has gone from being a primary school kid just going into the Juniors to taking her GCSEs. When I turned 40 I also qualified as a counsellor and started my own business, so I've also been self employed in what I consider to be a really important job to show up for, while trying to navigate a lot of extreme head pain. I'm not alone: in our mid-life, aren't we all doing a lot of stuff that's crucial? Like raising families, being really quite good in our careers and perhaps even rather high up, possibly looking after ageing parents too. It's the worst time for our hormones to have a punk rock phase, really.

I realised mine were getting out of hand one day back in 2015, when I was actually still only a sprightly 39. I woke up with a "headache" but I had really lovely plans that day with an old friend and I naively thought that having nice plans would mean I forgot about my head pain. I was driving over to hers and meeting her new baby, plus my 6 year old and her 5 year old were going to have a chance to play together.

My daughter and I made the half hour drive to her house, where I began to feel worse. The pain had gone from a niggling throb in my temple to a band of searing pain stretching over my whole left eyebrow. Still, I tried to concentrate on my friend's news – she'd just had a baby for crying out loud, I really wanted to hear all about it – and had a lovely cuddle with her newborn. My daughter and her son were playing a fantastic game of cars over in the corner of the room, and I was delighted to see them getting on so well, but every time one of them crashed something or made an appropriate car noise, the fire in my head intensified. I asked my friend for a glass of water, feeling sure I was just a bit dehydrated. The migraine laughed in my face. My friend asked me if I was OK, and I said I absolutely was. Internally, I was cheerleading myself to drive home, possibly stick my daughter in front of a film if I wasn't feeling better, and have a lie down.

I got my daughter strapped into her seat and set off down the road, heading out of my friend's village and towards the motorway I needed to be on to get home. The pain in my head was so intense, suddenly, that I knew I couldn't drive any further. My daughter picks up on everything and I didn't want to scare her (despite feeling quite scared myself by this point) so I pulled into a pretty village cul de sac where it was very quiet and shaded by trees, and suggested we have a snack before we get on the road. She was pleased by this new adventure and happily ate the biscuits I pulled out of my bag. Meanwhile, I grabbed my water bottle and chugged back a couple of paracetamol. That'll do it, I told myself. We'll just sit here for fifteen or twenty minutes and then I'll be good to go.

But I wasn't. The pain was making me feel quite unsteady. It was so hot and so sharp it was taking my breath away. It hurt to look up, just at normal things lit by daylight on a nice late spring day. Every time a car went by, or a bird chirruped, or my daughter exclaimed "Look Mummy, a ladybird!" the pain fizzed to an even higher crescendo. I felt so sick I began scanning the vicinity for the most suitable bush to throw up in, just in case. One thing was for sure: we weren't getting on a motorway right now. We just weren't.

Luckily, my friend lived only a mile or so away from my parents' house. I knew the route very well and it was a quiet road through one village and into the next. It wasn't ideal to be driving at all, but driving there was much safer than attempting to get back home, and even if my parents weren't in I had a key and I could sit quietly in their house while my daughter amused herself with the stash of toys and books they kept for her there. We set off, me having to come clean and admit I had "a bit of a headache" and that we'd just see if Nanna and Grandad were home so I could maybe have a bit more water.

My dad was home and, a migraine sufferer himself, knew immediately that I wasn't OK. He rooted some ibuprofen out of a drawer for me, gave me some water and told me to go and have a lie down in my old room: he was perfectly happy to get an unexpected playdate with his granddaughter. I collapsed gratefully into bed upstairs, drawing the curtains against the daylight and pressing the painful side of my head into the cool pillow. I felt certain that, having taken a double whammy of painkillers, I would be alright in no time. An hour, tops.

An hour passed. Dad came up to see if I needed anything. He could see I was really struggling and told me to stay put as long as I needed. I was so grateful to him but at the same time almost in tears of frustration: why wasn't anything working? Why wouldn't this pain just do one? How was I going to get home in time to cook dinner?

I rooted through my bag in desperation and unearthed some strong over the counter painkillers someone had recommended me for period pain. Sometimes I would have such mighty cramps that I would pass out. I'd learned to get these painkillers down me as soon as the cramps got bad enough to double me over and make me feel dizzy, and generally they would work to ease things enough that I didn't pass out. There were two left in the pack and although they contained paracetamol as well as their stronger ingredient, codeine, I literally couldn't do the maths in my head as to whether I'd taken the other paracetamol four hours ago or sooner. I mean, I'm not a mathematician, but I can subtract 4. Except, it turns out, when my head is having an invisible nail hammered into it. I took the painkillers. And gradually, gradually...the migraine didn't go, but it simmered down to a level I could be upright with. I didn't love the prospect of going out into daylight, never mind driving half an hour on the motorway, but I felt confident I could do it safely.

We reached home and I was grateful for my husband to take over care of both child and dinner. I was absolutely shattered, still in considerable pain and certainly not up for eating or doing much. It had been an ordeal but I felt comforted that at least now I was home, I could go to bed early and sleep it off. Tomorrow's a new day and all that...

Except it wasn't. I slept fitfully as the painkillers wore off and the pain returned. Come morning, the migraine was just as present and painful as it had been the day before. I was so dismayed: how long could this last? I'm not one to cancel plans and retreat to bed very easily, so I took some more painkillers and tried to swallow a bit of breakfast. I got through a day of friends visiting (including young children singing at full volume about poo) and childcare and did the bare minimum to keep our souls and house functioning. There followed another early night, and a better sleep, and the next day the migraine was almost gone. I felt like it was still throbbing away in one temple, but less insistently, and compared the the pain of the past 48 hours it felt quite manageable. I was terrified of it coming back full force, and drank enough water to fill a reservoir. I was also absolutely exhausted, feeling like I had a combination of sleep deprivation and a pretty bad hangover.

For the next three years, I had a migraine like this every two or three weeks. It wasn't ideal, and it felt like a big increase on the one or two a year that I'd had most of my life, but I knew it was perimenopause and I did my best to solve it with over the counter painkillers.

Then, the following year, two things happened at once: the migraines began coming far more frequently and my periods, always a handful, got much harder to manage.

Let's talk periods for a bit. They don't get enough airtime. When mine started at age 13, I found the volume of blood quite the challenge. "It might seem like a lot of blood," I remember reading in a book about periods, "but it's actually only half a teacup-full over the course of your whole period." Oh, really? Because if we are talking those teacups you *ride* in at Disneyland, then yeah, that might be about right.

As a teenager, I would bleed through a super flow tampon and a heavy duty sanitary pad in an hour. You can imagine what a bind that was at school. Luckily I was quite bolshy about it all and didn't baulk at asking to leave a lesson to use the loo with my backpack in tow, but even I crumbled the day I went to change my pad before PE only to discover blood had leaked all the way down my thighs. We had to wear hateful little shorts for PE and I was worried the no-nonsense PE teacher would make me play netball with all the blood on show. Nasty, plasticky school-issue toilet paper wasn't going to cut it in the clean up operation so I burst into tears and got sent home instead. And I can't tell you how many times I bled onto my bedding because I slept through for a few hours and didn't wake up to change my tampon and pad. I was forever ruining knickers and bedsheets.

Each period would be heavy like this for three or four days, before being a bit more reasonable and manageable for another four or five. I'd be glad to see the back of each one, but then it was less than three weeks before the whole thing would start over again.

I was told this was usual when starting periods (it's not) and that mine would settle down. And they did, sort of. I *only* had the heavy bleeding for two to three days, followed by a more regular seeming flow for four to five. But, by the time I was 17, the fainting started.

I had experienced period cramps before that point, as most women do. It was a hot, squeezing pain that came and went over the course of those heavy bleed days. But the first time I fainted I was at the end of my period, getting on with my day at sixth form, when I felt the cramps start up in a lesson. I thought it was a bit odd, but I'd come to expect periods to be a bit of a sod, so I assumed this was some new inconvenience I'd have to put up with. By break time, the cramps were so bad I was convinced my heavy flow must be back, and I rushed to the toilet with my bag to check. I had come on a little heavier, but nothing dramatic.

I had an anxious thought about tampons and toxic shock syndrome, and thought this new and increasingly sharp burning pain must mean something was terribly wrong. I decided not to put in a new tampon, and to just wear a pad for now. This was a needless fear: TSS isn't a concern as long as you are changing your tampon regularly, but tampons have always made cramps worse for me.

I went to find my friends near the canteen and tried to distract myself by chatting to them, but one of them said "Are you OK?" and another commented "You look really pale" and before I knew it, I was sliding down the wall in a faint. A PE teacher happened to be walking past and when I came round he was looking at me with great concern and an almost equal amount of fear. My friends were gathered round, and were picking up my bag and stuff. "It's my period," I managed to squeak. "Well I think we'd better send you home," said the PE teacher. He told me to take it very slowly and didn't let go my arm until he'd got me safely to the school office, with a friend carrying my bag and waiting with me until someone could pick me up. Weirdly, I felt fine by then, but it had shaken me up (possibly almost as much as that poor PE teacher) and I was glad to go home and take it easy.

There followed more than fifteen years of heavy periods with occasional fainting, always preceded by severe period cramps. I fainted at university, at home, at work (once in the middle of a meeting), while walking home from work, while walking home from the shops with my toddler (and having to panic-teach her how to call her dad on my mobile) and on my bike. I did get a year or two off after I had my daughter – having a baby did settle things down for a short while – but it was soon back to business as usual.

I did go to my GP about it. Once when I was a teenager, where it was recommended I take the combined oral contraceptive pill, which is commonly the first line in managing heavy, painful periods. However, there was some family history that made this type of pill a little more risky for me, so I ruled it out. I went back to see my GP in my twenties, when the pain and PMS got particularly bad for a while. I was prescribed mefenamic acid, which gave me diarrhoea. After a couple of days of managing horrible cramps, a gushing flow and explosive diarrhoea I decided it wasn't a combination I wanted in my life and never took the stuff again.

Fast forward to the perimenopause and my periods suddenly became worse. They were still pretty regular (once every 3 and a half weeks, lucky me) but they were suddenly heavier than ever, though thankfully no more painful. Instead of going through those super tampons and heavy duty towels in one hour, I was going through them in 45 minutes. Which made a difference. As a therapist, I work in 50 minute sessions, with a ten minute break between clients to take a breather, have a wee, maybe a quick cuppa and reset my head. If you're flooding into your clothes after 45 minutes, now you've got ten minutes to clean a chair, change your outfit, wash blood off yourself, change your tampon and towel, eat a biscuit because you feel wobbly and somehow be ready to see the next person who needs you.

And besides that, needing to be on a toilet every 45 minutes rules a lot of stuff out. Long car journey? Nope. Walk into town? Well, that takes 30 minutes BUT you'll bleed more heavily the more you move while upright, so probably not advisable. Pop to see a friend? Not unless they're a friend with a wipe clean sofa. Have a normal night's sleep? Oh dear me no. The flow will slow fractionally while you're lying down, but you will be up every couple of hours and you'd better sleep on an old beach towel unless you want a mattress that looks like it was central to a murder scene.

I tried a menstrual cup, since I had friends who reported those were great for allowing them to forget they were even on their period. One friend said she popped hers in in the morning and usually didn't need to empty it until the evening, when she'd wash it and pop it back in for bed. It would then comfortably last her all night long, allowing a blissful, uninterrupted night of sleep. A menstrual cup holds a lot more blood than a tampon and towel combined and it's perfectly safe to leave it in all day. I didn't hesitate to get one.

On the plus side, then: I could go four or five hours before it got full. A vast improvement. It felt comfortable in a way tampons don't always: sometimes they poke your cervix in a really irritating way and seem to make cramps worse. Plus, I could finally measure how much blood I was losing and know for sure that half a teacup thing was wildly out. I was losing 500ml per period, on average. Sometimes more like 750ml. I was filling enough teacups for a whole (admittedly gory and unconventional) tea party.

And the negative side of the menstrual cup, which ultimately consigned it to the back of my bathroom cabinet? Let's put it this way: have you seen The Shining?

OK, I'm exaggerating. A little. But getting a menstrual cup out of your vagina without spilling anything on yourself, your clothes, the toilet or the floor involves a deep squat and just the right combo of careful/firm tugging. Get it wrong and your bathroom or, so much worse, the toilet cubicle in your workplace/Marks and Spencer/the pub you went to for lunch is immediately transformed into a very convincing crime scene. Your knickers, trousers, shoes and socks will all be in the splash zone. If you are in your own bathroom at home, at least you can get changed and wash the blood off your hands and have a little cry while you wash out the menstrual cup. You can also wad as much loo roll between your legs as you need and waddle around bare from the waist down while you accomplish this. Imagine emerging from the toilet in a nice restaurant with a bloody menstrual cup in your blood stained hands, to attempt to clean everything in the shared sink. And while you are doing this, and nice members of the public give you a wide berth, you will still be gushing blood all over the gaff until you can get that newly washed cup back up your fanny.

So, for this reason, menstrual cups didn't free me up at all. I didn't feel I could cope with changing them anywhere except for in the privacy of my own bathroom, with full crime scene kit to hand.

So many things were just not possible during that first 2 or 3 days of my period, that I quite rightly got fed up and went to see my GP. She suggested the progesterone only pill (POP), which was more suitable for me given my family history, and as she tapped out the prescription on her computer she smiled and said "It may even stop your periods completely, you know, it does for about a third of women who take it." I thought that sounded too good to be true and, given the epic bleeding I'd always had, felt sure I'd be lucky to experience a reduction in flow. I picked up my prescription and hoped for the best.

Reader, I was period-free for the next three years. I hope I can convey to you some of the joy of those years (and that I continue to experience – now and then I come off it to see if I've gone through menopause yet, but at least that is at a time of my choosing and I can prepare in advance for the apocalypse). I hadn't really appreciated how much these massive bleeds every 25 days had weighed me down. I didn't realise until they were no longer a thing how much I had dreaded them, not to mention how much I had restricted myself while expecting them or having them.

On the POP I went swimming without a second thought, exercised for as long as I wanted, worked with my mind fully on my clients, sat on the whitest sofas and slept through every night. No bleeding, no cramps, no PMS. It was beautiful. It still is. God, I thought, no wonder women who have gone through the menopause talk about getting a new lease of life. It must be because they're cartwheeling through life period-free.

Unfortunately it wasn't such plain sailing on the migraine front. Just as the periods got heavier, the migraines got worse and more frequent. And, while the periods were immediately fixed by the POP, the migraines remained the same. Between 50% and 75% of my life was migraine.

I started keeping a diary, as I was sure I would find patterns that I could take to my GP, so that we could find a way forward. But quickly I realised there were no patterns. Where in the old days, migraines had hit me just before or during my period, now they had no rhyme or reason. Before I got myself on the POP, they would occur at literally any point in my natural cycle, sometimes not bothering me during my period at all but being awful the week before or the week afterwards. Sometimes they would last a day, other times they would last 3 days. Sometimes they would be on the left and sometimes on the right, usually in my temples and across one eyebrow, but sometimes causing pain in my neck and all over my head too. If I medicated, sometimes that would help and sometimes it would do nothing.

I read that it was best to get in as early as possible with medication. My instinct had been to "see how I go" and wait for it to get quite bad before I would take something, so I stopped doing that and had a paracetamol as soon as I felt the early gnawing sensations. Sometimes that stopped it in its tracks and I could only guess at how bad an attack I had prevented. Sometimes that worked for a few hours and I would get the pain back a bit later. And other times it would do nothing, like chucking a glass of water on a house fire, and I may as well not have bothered.

That was when I would roll out the big guns and take my period pain tablets, which contained paracetamol and codeine. Often, in those early days, that would do the trick. It was like a magic button. I'd take the paracetamol-codeine combo (always making sure to leave four hours since the paracetamol I'd tried initially), if possible have a lie down, and start to feel the pain subsiding within half an hour. A lovely relaxed sort of feeling would wash over me thanks to the codeine as well, which would have the effect of making me realise I had been tensing all my muscles against the pain and now no longer needed to.

My migraines made me feel sick, but I have to say I am lucky in this respect. I have only actually thrown up on half a dozen occasions from migraine pain. I know some of my fellow migraineurs are way more nauseated and vomit copiously during attacks, unable to even keep water down. For me, the nausea has been exactly like pregnancy nausea, which I was also fortunate with. It isn't a nice feeling, but you know you're not actually going to vomit, and counter-intuitively having sips of water or a little something to eat actually makes it disappear for a while.

One thing I wasn't expecting was how migraines changed my cognitive processes. The attentive reader will have picked up on my tendency towards the dramatic. I like to think I normally keep this in check. However, during a migraine I have frequently believed whole-heartedly that something in my brain is going to burst and I am going to die. I felt frightened to look in the mirror during one migraine attack because I was absolutely certain that my eye was full of blood (it wasn't. Full of sad little tears maybe).

On a smaller scale, I also become very forgetful, completely unable to follow simple instructions, very impatient, a bit depressed, more anxious and a bit fixated on things.

And I get earworms. You know you sometimes get a song stuck in your head for a bit? I got a song that I really hated stuck in there for two whole weeks. Migraines came and went around it. I still get nervous anytime I hear it (it's a popular song from the 2000s that still gets a fair amount of radio play. I wouldn't have minded had it been Iron Maiden).

I also feel very fortunate that I don't experience the aura that many migraine sufferers describe. I don't suffer from any visual disturbances (although I do become much less able to tolerate light of any kind) or hear ringing in my ears or anything like that. The closest I came to an aura was smelling something that wasn't there for a few days before the pain of the migraine arrived. I was baffled as to why my family couldn't smell the awful thing that one of the cats had surely brought in and hidden and that I couldn't find the source of despite going all over the house. Then I realised I could still smell the horror when I went outside, and it dawned on me that it was all in my head. It's only happened a couple of times but I did wonder why it couldn't be a lovely aroma of rose petals or a subtle sandalwood scent.

So, migraine was keeping me guessing, never being quite the same or responding in quite the same way each time, but I decided I had to take this to my GP and see what he thought about it. It was getting harder to ride them out and I found myself more frequently unable to work or do the things I would normally do at home.

My GP was very kind and understanding, and really clued up about perimenopause. I know this is not everyone's experience, so I felt very lucky. He listened to my tales of migraine lottery and looked through the colourful migraine diary I presented him with, and suggested prescribing a triptan. Triptans are a relatively new migraine treatment (they first appeared in the 1990s) that work by changing how blood circulates in your brain and how your brain processes pain signals[x]. They are not painkillers but they can stop the pain of a migraine attack very quickly. The snag is that you can't take any more than 2 per week or 6 per month.

Therefore, hearing how codeine had helped me with the worst of the pain, my GP prescribed some codeine to use at other times. He was careful to say I shouldn't take too much of that, either: it can be addictive (and it was easy to see why – that gentle, relaxed feeling it produced was pleasant, though I wouldn't swap it for a clear head if I was feeling well). He said I was right to try simple medication like paracetamol as a first resort, and said I could usefully try ibuprofen instead or as well. Ibuprofen, he explained, is anti-inflammatory, and migraines are caused by a nerve-controlled inflammation of the membrane between the brain and the skull[xi].

I went off to try these new strategies and note down the results in my ever growing migraine diary. I got plenty of data as the episodes came thick and fast. Ibuprofen had roughly the same success rate as paracetamol: sometimes it seemed to vanish a threatened migraine before it even got hold, other times it was like a fart in a blizzard. The triptan had no impact at all. It tasted rank going down and almost caused me to throw up on the spot. I thought: this better be worth it. I waited. Nothing happened. I was gutted after all I'd heard about the miracle of triptans. The codeine continued to be my secret weapon. When other things had failed, I took it, and it made me feel much better very quickly. It lasted, too: once I'd taken it, the migraine would usually not come back that day. I carried codeine everywhere with me.

I didn't leave it too long before visiting my GP again, because migraine was still a frequent life feature. I had booked in to see him, and a day or so before I got one of the worst migraines I've ever had. I was in so much pain that I couldn't work, I couldn't even open my eyes. Every time I did it felt like a knife was being driven into my eyeball and a red hot poker was being run into the brain tissue behind it (cognitive larks again). I had run through the sequence of taking ibuprofen, then codeine, then out of desperation a triptan, and nothing had worked at all. Not even to take the edge off a bit. I was lying on my bed, clutching my eye and the side of my head, whimpering, and my husband was quite worried about me. "Shall I call the GP and see if he can see you today?" he suggested reasonably. I just had a little cry. I couldn't find words to answer him.

An hour later I was loaded into the car with dark glasses on, clutching a sick bag. My daughter, now ten years old, had got home from school and was helping her dad get me to the surgery, which is a ten minute walk from our house. Normally I'd think nothing of going on foot, but walking in daylight with normal street noises assaulting me genuinely felt like an impossible task. As it was, I hung onto both of them as they manoeuvred me into the waiting room, and then sat as still as possible with my eyes shut behind my dark glasses, almost unable to breathe through the pain. When my GP saw me, pale, shaky and accessorising with a sick bag, he knew well enough what was going on. He took my blood pressure and said very gently "That's really pretty good, considering" and proceeded to ask me, in a mercifully quiet voice, lots of questions about what I'd been experiencing and what I'd tried. It was very useful to have another adult there, to answer the complicated stuff like "And what time did you take the triptan?" and to help me absorb the advice he was about to offer. Remembering important information while migraining is like trying to thread a needle while wearing oven gloves.

"I think you need to stop taking the codeine," he said.

But...but...I had been careful not to take too much (was three or four times a week too much? Sometimes that did mean three or four days in a row) and never to take it unless paracetamol or ibuprofen had failed. Was he worried I was becoming an addict?

"What I'm really worried about is that the codeine might be making your migraines worse," he explained.

But...but...they were the only damn thing that worked for me! How could that be true?

I understood better later, when my brain was functioning again. Our brains don't like too much pain (fair enough) or, conversely, too much pleasure. They actually prefer to be in a nice, neutral sort of balance where things are quite middling. So, when a migraine hits, the brain goes into panic mode. This is a lot of pain, it thinks, and we are a long way off balance. Along comes the codeine and, wham! In a short space of time, the brain is not only no longer in pain but it has tipped over into the realm of feeling a fair whack of pleasure (remember that lovely, relaxed feeling codeine bestows?) Now the brain is aware that it's on a kind of high, and that can't be maintained, so it'd better do something to try to redress the balance. Sometimes, the way it attempts that is to produce more pain, sort of failing to stop in the neutral zone and overcompensating until it's back in the pain zone again.

I also held a personal theory that, because codeine feels quite nice, and yet I don't feel any temptation to take it on days when I'm well, might a naughty little addiction pixie in my brain somewhere create some sort of migraine pain to get me to take some more? I don't have any medical science to back up my addition pixie theory, I just thought it might explain the increase in migraines.

Anyway, it made sense to me that I needed to try to manage without codeine, though that was an almighty blow. I'd leaned on it a lot. And while I wasn't taking anything like the amount considered problematic by doctors, or even close to the maximum amount stipulated on the back of the box, everyone's body is different. Mine seemed to respond quite well to codeine, on the one hand – it took away my migraines so efficiently. But maybe that meant I was also more sensitive than the average person to taking too much, and my threshold would be lower.

My GP had suggested that, instead of treating the migraines with painkillers, we try preventing them in the first place. He offered HRT initially, as we knew the migraines were connected to perimenopause, and that was the logical first line of defence. However, it would mean I'd have to come off the POP and my periods would return.

"Erm...anything else I can try?"

The next line of defence was to try amitriptyline, a medication commonly prescribed at higher doses to treat anxiety and depression.

"But I'm not anxious or depressed," I pointed out, "how will it work for me?"

"Well, it changes how much of a chemical called serotonin is available in your brain," my GP explained, "and one of the things that can influence is how your nerves receive pain signals. It might mean you experience less migraine pain."

I was familiar with how antidepressants worked from my job of course, but also from an episode of depression I suffered myself some twenty years back. It seemed quite reasonable that it might be worth a try. As with taking these things for depression and anxiety, it's important to give them a chance to get into your system – a good six weeks is usually long enough to see some improvement if there is going to be any. In the meantime, I was strictly limited to conservative paracetamol and ibuprofen use.

"I mean, I suppose I do experience a bit of anxiety, just about the migraines themselves," I said, almost as an afterthought.

"That can be another reason that the amitriptyline is helpful," he said.

"But...if I didn't have the migraines, there wouldn't be any anxiety, so how have I gotten into this mess?"

He just gave me a sympathetic look.

I'm not going to sugar coat it. The next couple of months were hellish.

I was determined to get the best out of this new approach as possible, so I didn't take paracetamol or ibuprofen at all, and I realised how often they had been preventing an absolute beast of a migraine from ever arriving. I also didn't take any codeine, so I had no way of damping down the really bad migraines.

I tried whenever I could to keep going, but sometimes I just knew I wouldn't be able to concentrate at work and give a client the full attention they should get, and I had to cancel their session. This didn't feel great at all. Longer term clients understood, and I could often rearrange their session and work more hours on another day. Newer clients understandably sometimes didn't come back. And I began to hesitate to take new clients on. Every counsellor has a supervisor, who they meet with once a month and who helps ensure they are doing OK and patiently assists with unknotting any tricky problems. Mine was very worried about me and was suggesting that cutting my workload would be a good idea. But I hated the very thought: I'd only qualified for this career that I turned out to love a couple of years earlier. I didn't want to slow down.

But in order to cancel as little work as possible, I began cancelling social stuff. A late night would make me more vulnerable to a migraine. Driving made me more vulnerable, too. All of my friends got used to me flaking on them during this time. They are lovely: they forgave me. But it didn't feel like a great compromise.

Nor did ducking out on family stuff all the time. My husband has cheerfully taken the reins so many times when I pushed myself at work only to find I had nothing left over for family. Again, it didn't feel good at all, but I didn't know what else to do.

The amitriptyline made me feel tired, one of the most common side effects. I mean, migraine makes you feel tired, so I was quite prepared to swap tiredness caused by migraine for tiredness caused by amitriptyline. But as six weeks dragged into eight and then on into twelve, I was seeing no benefit. I was putting up with all this pain, cancelling my life left right and centre, and if I was supposed to not be feeling anxious about that any more...well, let's just say the amitriptyline was definitely not for me.

I went back to the GP. He admitted he'd started me off on the lowest possible dose of amitriptyline, and that if he bumped it up a bit I'd probably start noticing a difference. He also slung in a different triptan. There's a whole family of those and, while the first one I'd tried hadn't worked for me, one of its siblings might.

It was coming up to Christmas and, as always, we were hosting a house full of relatives. I liked hosting. I like to cook and the jolly chaos of it all for one day is usually fun. But naturally I was on day 3 of a rough migraine by the time that Christmas rolled around. The paracetamol hadn't worked. The ibuprofen hadn't worked. The new triptan hadn't worked. I caved and took two codeine (over-the-counter ones since I wasn't being prescribed any more – so they were half the strength of my prescription tablets). Within the hour, I felt like myself again. OK, myself on a candyfloss cloud. But Christmas went brilliantly, and I really enjoyed it.

I did stick with the amitriptyline for another three months, and did without painkillers. The amitriptyline never did anything for me except make me more tired, but going without pain relief did teach me one big lesson. I was surprised at how much I could do while in pain.

I don't think I've ever been particularly stoic about pain and, if anything, I probably feel pain more readily than I think some other people do. Migraine pain can be severe enough to make your body think there is an emergency: it does useful crisis response stuff like shutting down luxury functions such as digestion and rational thought, and puts you into fight or flight mode, flooding you with adrenaline and, when the pain doesn't go away quickly enough, raising cortisol levels[xii]. While that isn't pleasant, it can be used to achieve things you thought your migraine would surely prevent you from doing.

For example, one afternoon during this time when I was feeling spectacularly bad, my daughter received a gift of two badminton racquets and a pack of shuttlecocks and was desperate to go out into the garden and play with them. By this era of my migraine career I had stopped telling my nearest and dearest every time I had a migraine, because it was so often that I felt like a broken record. So as she bounced around the garden with her badminton racquet, excited for me to join in, I decided not to say no. I wondered what would happen if I just went out there and rebelled against my body and my throbbing head and just smashed a game of garden badminton. Perhaps I would pass out – it seemed likely, but at least I'd have a soft landing on the grass. Perhaps I would throw up – I'm such a bad gardener no one would notice. My daughter would definitely be more happy, and that felt like the more important thing at that moment. I was so heartily sick of migraine stopping me from doing stuff. I put on dark glasses and went out there.

I didn't throw up or pass out. The pain was blinding, but then it had been before. I missed every last shuttlecock, but that made my daughter laugh. She was better at this than me! I felt like I was only half there – but I was there. I didn't think about how long I could keep it up or what else I had to do that day, I just put one foot in front of the other and kept waving a racquet around, and it was alright.

I started applying that to everything. Going to work didn't make things worse. Mainly my job is to sit quietly and listen to people, and if I am a bit slower than usual they just get to say more and get fewer of my questions – which doesn't seem to do them any harm. Sometimes they need to have a good shout or rant and admittedly those are harder sessions with a migraine, but most often I am OK to be there, and I am so glad I was. I felt a lot better being at work with pain than I felt cancelling work and going to bed.

I realise that continuing work was only possible because of the nature of the job I do. If I'd been a teacher or a driver or a doctor or worked in a shop or an office, I wouldn't have been able to work through a migraine. In most jobs, I would have had to take so many sick days that I would have been fired. In most self-run businesses, the business would have folded. So you are allowed to want to slap me for being fortunate enough to have a job I feel I can do in pain.

Doing something quiet with friends or family didn't make things worse. Neither did a walk in the fresh air with dark glasses on and earplugs in. Neither did reading a book (reading a screen definitely makes things worse: I still avoid that when I have a migraine).

Going out somewhere noisy was a fairly obvious no-no, as was driving a car. I never did that either with a migraine or when taking codeine: I know my reaction times would not be as sharp and I'd feel terrible if anything happened.

This felt like a step forward with the migraines: nothing had changed them yet, but I had shifted my own position relating to them a little bit. In therapy, we're always harking back to that notion like annoying little bitches – "If you can't change the situation, change your outlook" – but there is truth in it. It is very helpful to be able to accept situations you are stuck with, because it takes down your stress response if you are not constantly fighting it.

I did go back to my GP though, and we agreed I'd given the amitriptyline a decent shot.

"Let's try you on beta blockers," he said brightly.

"Aren't those for people with heart conditions?" I asked.

"Well, often, yes," he explained, "but they're useful for migraine too. They can block the impact of adrenaline and improve the flow of blood through your veins. Sometimes migraine is caused by blood vessels widening too much and the beta blocker will keep that in check."

I mean, I had felt like my adrenaline was going nuts sometimes because of the migraines, so maybe this was just the ticket.

"How are you getting on with that triptan?" he checked.

"Oh, it doesn't seem to work on me."

"Well, I did start you off on - "

"The lowest possible dose? Yeah, I've noticed that's a pattern with you."

"Well, we could try it at a higher dose, see if that helps when you have an attack."

"I'm game."

I began the beta blockers right away, and felt cautiously optimistic. After a few weeks, I did notice a bit of an improvement. Nothing dramatic: migraines were now 35% of my life instead of 50%. But I would take that. It was still progress. They were still as bad when they came, but this new higher dose of triptan worked pretty well. I took it (tried not to gag: they all seem to taste revolting) and while its effects would not be as quick as the codeine, within one to two hours I would be feeling significantly, and sometimes completely, better. The migraine would rush back in after 6 or 7 hours – I guess that was the triptan wearing off – but it gave me 6 grace periods a month.

The new challenge then was figuring out in advance which six days of the month I wanted to save my triptans for. Should I prioritise them to ensure I was fit for work, or save them up for social occasions I didn't want to miss? I found it too complex to work out how many I'd had in a rolling month, so I went by calendar month, and at the start of each would try to weigh up what I might most need them for.

It took a while to get it right, but my priorities went roughly like this:

1. Days when I will be parenting solo because my husband is out of town.

2. Days when something lovely and special is happening, like a holiday, birthday, day out, trip etc.

3. Days when I am required to drive somewhere and it would be bloody inconvenient if we had to walk or take public transport instead.

I would always run out of triptan allocation by priority 3, and not to sound boastful about my social life because I promise it's just an average one, but often by priority 2. Therefore triptans never got used just to get to work (I just managed working with pain) or for everyday stuff.

Of course, if I didn't happen to have a migraine on the day I'd reserved a triptan for, that triptan could in theory be used on another occasion. But in reality, I bought into the scarcity mentality and always thought "I'd better save them, just in case." As a result, I rarely take all six in a month. But whenever I took them, I was grateful for the few hours off and for the break that provided. Doing stuff while in pain is possible, but it does take it out of you.

So I reported back to my GP that things were going rather well. He wasn't as enthusiastic about the 35% migraine rate as I was ("I'd like to get it lower than that," he said. Yeah, me too!) but I was reluctant to take him up on his suggestion that we increase the beta blocker dose. One common side effect of beta blockers is that they make you tired. They slow your heart rate so I was finding mine was down in the 50s rather than up in the 70s or 80s like usual, and that did tend to make me sleepy whenever I sat down for too long. I was alright at work, when I had a client needing my full attention, but if I sat down to watch something nice on TV, I'd rarely see the end of it. I had to stop going to the cinema because, despite the film being incredibly exciting, I would not be able to fight off sleep in those amazing recliner seats.

However, turning into a total granny about naps was acceptable to me if my migraines were going to be fewer and I was getting bigger breaks to recover between them. Except that stopped happening as soon as it had started. I had maybe a couple of months at 35% and then I ramped up again to 50% and beyond. I was back to square one.

My GP heard all about it of course. He was very attentive and sympathetic. "Maybe this is just your hormone fluctuations," he suggested, quite reasonably, "are you sure you don't want to come off the pill and try HRT?"

It so happened that right at that stage of things, over in non migraine life, we were about to go and live and work abroad for a bit. I was already worried about managing without my understanding GP, and navigating a new adventure whilst coping with migraine. I didn't think putting heavy unmanageable periods back into the mix was wise. I said I'd persevere with the beta blockers, keep the triptans handy, and see how things went.

To give you the short version, living abroad didn't quite go as planned. The schooling arrangements didn't work out as we hoped and Plan B involved a school much further away, which I had to get my daughter to on public transport. This meant I couldn't work full time, and part time working wasn't really a thing where we lived. Without a job, I had no medical insurance, and doctor's appointments were costly. A very wise part of me had packed a few packets of OTC paracetamol and codeine as well as some OTC ibuprofen and codeine. When my beta blockers ran out, I realised for sure that they hadn't really cut down the migraines. I had the same roughly 50%-75% rate. I started taking the painkillers from home as and when I needed them, and it really helped. I got a family member to bring more from the UK when they visited. I rationed them carefully – I had never taken huge amounts of them anyway – because I wasn't sure whether you could get them in the (non English speaking) country we were in nor how I would begin to ask for them.

Interestingly, on a short hop over to a country that shall remain nameless for a long weekend away, I walked into a pharmacy to purchase a Calpol equivalent for my daughter and the pharmacist, unprompted, offered me Valium. So I probably could have got anything I wanted with a bit of nerve. I am just genuinely not that daring.

Once we were back in the UK again, there was a pandemic to contend with, and I couldn't bring myself to book a GP appointment to discuss something as routine as migraine when people were dying all over the show, so I continued with my regime of painkillers. It worked well sometimes, and less well other times. The paracetamol and ibuprofen were as hit and miss as ever. I had read something about soluble aspirin being worth a try as it gets into your system a bit faster, so I experimented with that. Again, sometimes it worked like a charm, and other times I may as well have not bothered.

My magic bullet, codeine, was becoming similarly unreliable. Sometimes I swallowed it and was like "What migraine?" and other times it just took it down a notch. Increasingly, it didn't work. Occasionally, it seemed to make the pain worse, although I was never sure if it was just doing nothing and the pain increase was the natural course of a worsening migraine.

It became unreliable enough that, come mid 2021, I decided it was time to have another chat with my GP. I'd done my reading, and I knew there were three main things to try for migraine prevention, aside from the HRT. As well as amitriptyline and beta blockers, neither of which had worked for me, there were anticonvulsants, usually prescribed for epileptics. Usually Topiramate is prescribed, which works by decreasing the electrical activity in the brain. In epileptics this can help prevent seizures, but in migraine sufferers it can restore the balance of nerve activity in the brain.

Unfortunately for me, but fortunately for the rest of the UK, my GP was off somewhere contributing to the Covid vaccination effort. I saw another GP – and when I say "saw" I mean I had a phonecall with him – and he really made me miss my regular GP.

After attempting to tell me, at the ripe old age of 46, that I was too young for menopause (don't worry, I enlightened him about perimenopause, but I suspect this didn't warm him to me any) he informed me that my migraines were probably due to stress. I mean, I did feel quite stressed at that moment, having someone who'd spoken to me on the phone for three minutes concluding that he'd explained the migraine issues I'd been having for some five years. But I put that aside and told him that the one thing his much more empathic colleague and I hadn't tried was Topiramate.

"Well I'm not prescribing that for you."

"Can I ask why not?" I knew it had some unpleasant side effects for some people. Maybe he was concerned about me.

"It's too unusual."

"I'm sorry?"

"It's not usual to prescribe it for migraine prevention."

"It's all over the internet that there are three main prevention medications and this is one of them." (Doctors *really* love you if you attempt to contradict them with something you read on the internet.)

"I'm telling you it's too unusual and I am not prescribing it."

Yikes. It was upsetting. I waited six months until my regular GP was back and tried having the same conversation with him.

"What do you think about me trying Topiramate?" I said.

"I think we need to try that next, yes," he agreed.

Thankfully, Topiramate didn't come with any side effects for me. Not even tiredness, folks! However, nor did it impact the frequency or severity of my migraines in any way, so not really a big win. I gave it a shot for six months, but had to admit defeat.

So, what next? I'd tried everything. I still wasn't keen to try HRT. I'd come off my POP to see what a natural period was like, three years on. It was absolutely horrendous. I went straight back on the POP again. My thought process was: I have learned a few things about living with migraines. They do limit my life, but I've got it down to a sort of acceptable minimum. Heavy periods feel less easy to work with: I think I am more limited by them. Do I want migraine up to 50% of the time or heavy bleeding 30-40% of the time (assuming a bleed lasting 7-10 days every 25 days)? I know the answer might very well be different for someone else, but I chose to keep the migraines over the periods. My decision was also influenced by HRT not having a great track record for helping with migraines; it tends to make little difference[xiii].

For the past three years, that's how I've managed. Always trying paracetamol, ibuprofen or soluble aspirin first (I generally choose one at random, none of them seem to have a success rate better than the others) and then turning to my OTC codeine mixed with either paracetamol or ibuprofen. If I took paracetamol initially, then I will choose the codeine with ibuprofen, so as not to take too much paracetamol. And if I picked the ibuprofen first, I'll take the codeine with paracetamol, in order not to overdo the ibuprofen. With any drug of the same type, it's important to leave at least four hours between doses, and to always follow any other instructions on the packet or given to you by a pharmacist or doctor.

The exception to this is if it's a designated triptan day, OR I have a triptan allowance left because we're near the end of the month and I've hardly used them, and the above regime has let me down and I'm a bit desperate. It's a ride-by-the-seat-of-your-pants and make-it-up-as-you-go-along kind of a system, but it's the best I've got.

Sometimes, and always on about day 3 or 4 of a migraine, I convince myself I've become addicted to codeine and brought this all on myself. At that point, I hand my migraine diary to my husband, and he says something like "Well, you've only taken two codeine, one today and one yesterday, and you've only had one dose of ibuprofen and an aspirin besides that. Are you sure you shouldn't be taking something else?"

And now, at last, at the lofty old age of 49, I'm seeing my migraine frequency start to come down the other side of the mountain. It's been more than a couple of months (more like six) so I hope it's not just a fluctuation in hormones. I hope it means I'm nearing menopause itself, that mythical date in the calendar when periods might become a thing of the past, with migraines consigned to the bin at the same time.

Which of course they may not be. I may go back to having a couple of migraines a year. I may remain where I am, having a migraine for 10% of the rest of my life. But I'm really hoping they do one and I get to forget what they're like, just like I knew nothing of this horror before my periods began.

Case studies

I work with a great variety of people and they bring all kinds of concerns into the therapy room. Often therapy is a complex process with many threads, and my favourite kind of work is when I really get the opportunity to know multiple aspects of someone and how their challenges interconnect. This tends to lead to a depth of work that best serves the client and feels like a helpful collaboration between us.

It would be unusual to "just" see someone for migraine management, though that would be absolutely welcome. More often, I have seen clients struggle with perimenopausal migraines as part and parcel of a larger picture, which I think is probably common.

The case studies here are heavily disguised to protect privacy and maintain confidentiality. They are composites of several clients, and all personal or identifying details have been changed.

Anita – finding ways to manage stress and guilt

Anita began therapy with me when she was approaching her fiftieth birthday. It's not unusual for people to begin therapy shortly before or after a big milestone birthday or event, and for Anita turning fifty was causing her to think through where she was in her life and where she wanted to be.

She began by apologising, and listing all the ways in which she felt she should be grateful for her lot. She was married to a lovely man, they'd been together for 30 years, and they had two teenage daughters who were thriving in their studies. She enjoyed her job, managing a large fundraising department for a branch of a well known charity, and looked forward to regular breaks when she and husband retreated to a cottage they'd recently bought in the Lakes, their favourite place to go walking.

The problem, then, was these migraines, the first of which had hit her "like a tonne of bricks" just two years previously. She had been so floored by the sudden onset of pain and so scared by its relentless throbbing through one side of her head for the next 48 hours that she ended up sobbing on the phone to 111, afraid that she was suffering from a tumour. Surely she couldn't be in this much pain and there be nothing seriously wrong with her? Her husband Googled her symptoms (pain on one side, nausea, having to stay in a dark room, feeling worse if she moved) and reassured her it sounded like migraine. He brought her water and paracetamol and although nothing relieved the pain, she was comforted by his presence, and grateful for him taking over all the household duties as well as calling her team at work to let them know she wouldn't be in.

She visited her GP once she was feeling better and the GP thought this very likely to be a perimenopausal migraine. Anita knew she had been in perimenopause for some time, because she'd had hot flushes and night sweats on and off since her early forties, but previously she'd felt fortunate that those were her only symptoms. While the hot flushes and night sweats hadn't been fun, disrupting her sleep and causing embarrassment at work sometimes, the migraines seemed so much worse. The GP warned Anita that she might get more of them now, and possibly for the next few years, and to come back if she wanted to discuss more treatment options.

Anita went back to work and back to her life and kept her fingers crossed that it had just been a one off. After all, she had never suffered from migraine before. But just ten days later, she felt a warning throb in her temple in the middle of a big meeting, and was overcome by dread. She tried to keep the meeting going – very quietly taking a paracetamol from her handbag while someone else was giving a presentation, and draining her water bottle – but soon found the overhead lights and even the normal noise of colleagues discussing proposals was far too much. She excused herself and threw up in the toilets.

She felt dizzy and disorientated as well as hardly knowing what to do with herself for the pain. It was astonishing to her how rapidly it had escalated. She had to ask a colleague to call her husband to come and collect her – there was no way she could have driven home. Again, she was completely out of action for 48 hours, unable to get up except to use the bathroom, unable to sleep except in snatches, unable to eat and unable to tolerate much light or sound.

The worst of this, for Anita, was that this one had hit a weekend, and on weekends she always went to see her mother, who lived an hour away and was quite frail. Anita would typically arrive on a Saturday lunchtime, take her mother out to the supermarket for her groceries, take her out for lunch, and then return to her bungalow to do any jobs she needed taking care of. There were things she needed every week, like changing her bedsheets and sorting out her medication into a manageable daily pill dispenser, and then there were often random things like needing the lawn mowed or the sticky cupboard door fixed. Anita would fly round with a hoover or don her rubber gloves, while her mother chatted about who she'd seen from the neighbourhood that week or what was on the telly. And although it was hard work and took up a sizeable chunk of her weekend, to Anita it felt like she was able to give her mother some care back, as she'd cared for her when she was a child.

Until she couldn't. She began getting migraines with alarming frequency, meaning she would miss as many as one weekend visit out of two with her mother, and when she was able to make it she worried about an attack coming while she was there and how she would get herself home. Not to mention how much she knew her mother would worry if she witnessed Anita in the throes of an attack, when she really was quite incapacitated. She was afraid of putting them both through that.

She felt incredibly guilty about these missed visits. Also, because it was genuinely hard for her mother to manage without the help, she found herself going over on a weekday evening, often shortly after a migraine had cleared when she seemed to find herself extra tired. Usually she was also catching up on whatever else she had missed at home and at work, too, so those post-migraine days felt especially hectic. She felt real pressure to be there for her mother, her husband and daughters and to continue being the up-to-speed boss she usually was in her working life. But it just wasn't possible to do it all.

It was interesting to watch how feeling guilty about her regular incapacitation kept her in a loop of shame that prevented her from working out what to do. She would feel guilty for what she'd missed through illness, and that was unbearable, so the moment she started to feel better she would leap back into action again in all her roles, attempting to "make up for" her absence. In doing so, she would overstretch herself when really she needed more recovery time, and sometimes exhaust herself further. Sometimes, this would even bring a new migraine surging in just a few days later, and the cycle would begin all over again. Anita had to miss therapy sessions when she had a migraine but, even allowing for the missed sessions, it took us a while to move from the overwhelming sense of guilt and shame to finding a space to reflect on what to do.

Guilt felt for things we cannot help is terribly difficult to shift. If Anita had felt guilty because she had chosen not to visit her mother, because she wanted to go away with her husband say, then feeling might have turned into action. Along the lines of "I do feel guilty that I didn't see Mum last weekend when I went away, so I'll stay a couple of extra hours next Saturday." When we can own it, we can work with it. However, when Anita felt guilty because of her migraine, which obviously wasn't under her control, she got trapped as the guilt turned to shame. This can go along the lines of "If I was stronger I'd be able to carry on" or "It must be my fault for not managing well enough." It's hard to work with those sorts of feelings, because they can tend to lodge in the core of us and make us feel that we ourselves are bad or inadequate.

Gradually and gently, we began to look at how while the migraines were not under Anita's control, some aspects of managing them might be. Her first step was to go back to her GP and fill her in on what had been happening since she first visited. The GP was able to talk through some choices with Anita for preventing and treating her migraines. After discussing her options, Anita decided to try HRT as a preventative measure. Her GP explained that while HRT hasn't really been proven to help prevent perimenopausal migraine, it often is effective at controlling hot flushes and night sweats, both of which can trigger migraine. She also prescribed her a triptan to try when an attack arrived, and explained how this might stop a migraine in its tracks.

While a sympathetic GP and appropriate medication was part of the plan, Anita and I started to look at what else she could do to feel better. She recognised that she was feeling a lot of dread: dread for the next migraine arriving and derailing either a visit that made such a huge difference to her mother or something big at work. She'd even missed university open days with her eldest daughter, and couldn't attend a concert her youngest was playing in – there always seemed to be something she desperately didn't want a migraine to ruin, yet inevitably it did.

We began to do some contingency planning. In the event of a migraine, who else could step in to look after her mother? Anita had no siblings, so we looked into other options. Sometimes her husband could go in her place, as their daughters were increasingly independent and could manage perfectly well parent-free for part of a weekend. There was also a good neighbour of her mother's, who was recently widowed and often popped in for a coffee: it turned out that she was more than willing to stand in for Anita some weekends, and was quite adept at managing the medications and the household tasks. Anita also got in touch with a local care agency, who arranged to be on call to provide care if family or neighbours couldn't. That was a slightly more pricey option, but it felt worth it to know she could pay them to show up if needed. She filed a list of things her mother would need in her absence with the agency – which medications, where to find clean linen, how to reset the boiler, etc – so that she wouldn't have to try to give detailed sets of instructions if she was ill. This cheat sheet was so useful that she gave her husband and the neighbour a copy, too. It helped her massively to know she'd got people to step in who would be able to manage.

She had always been adamant that she didn't want anything at work to change, because she had always loved her job, and she had worked hard through bringing up two children to hold onto her career and reach the management position she had coveted and was good at. She admitted that she had dreams about being "let off" work and feeling immense relief that she didn't have to keep up the fast pace – something she'd found challenging but exciting before migraines, and impossible now. But if she let herself off work – we explored ideas around taking some time out or doing a different role – she'd lose everything she'd worked so hard for, and that seemed unfair.

Eventually she came to accept that by continuing to work as hard as she did, she might find migraines more of a struggle. It was harder to concede time to them and it was tougher to come back and hit the ground running when they were over. But if that was better than giving up her job, then that was what she was choosing.

Until she came in for a session one day with her eyes twinkling. I could tell this was not a migraine day for her, nor was she in a postdrome: I had come to observe what those looked like. She had a bounce to her even as she took her seat and told me "I think I've found the solution." After a chance lunch catch up with the manager of another regional branch, she'd heard about a deputy manager from his office who was on the verge of leaving because she was struggling to balance work with caring for her terminally ill partner. This deputy had asked to go part time initially, but the request had been refused, as their region was painfully short staffed. It turned out that she was happy to travel to Anita's branch and take on a management role two days a week, allowing her some respite from her partner's care and a hopeful step up her own career ladder which might stand her in good stead for her uncertain future. Meanwhile, Anita would continue in her role for the other three days as best she could. No one could know for sure how long the job share arrangement would last, since the woman with the terminally ill partner had a very uncertain timeline, but it seemed worth a try.

The arrangement ended up stretching for more than three years, and it was "a game changer", as Anita put it herself. Having three days to cover rather than five gave her so much more leeway. If she was hit by a migraine on "her" days, it was often an option to catch up on her non-working weekdays when she felt better. Not having all the management responsibility also meant she didn't feel it was all down to her. Seeing how well her new job share settled into the role encouraged her to give a few more responsibilities to their deputies and see how they got on. The load was better shared and while she did eventually return to full time management, she never took back all the work that had once been on her to do list.

Unfortunately HRT didn't help with Anita's migraines. She continued to take it because it did help with the hot flushes and night sweats, and Anita had done a lot of research into some of the benefits of HRT on bone density. And although the first triptan she tried didn't help, the second one she tried did, and she was able to plan which days to take them on if a migraine hit. It meant she missed far fewer Saturdays with her mother, and she often had enough left over to ensure she didn't miss things that were important to her. It wasn't a perfect system, and she still had times when she couldn't function. But it was better than it had been, and it made her feel that she had some degree of agency over the migraines.

Funnily enough, the second triptan being so effective helped dissolve a lot of the guilt and shame she felt about being incapacitated by migraine. She told me: "The fact that I can just take this little pill and the pain subsides – it's not quite instant, but I actually feel it ebbing away within twenty minutes or so – it means I really do have migraines."

"Well, of course you do – there was some doubt there before?" I asked.

"Yes, I didn't realise how little I believed myself. I would lay there, unable to move in the dark, and think to myself *come on Anita, buck yourself up, it can't be that bad!* And yet, taking this triptan and so quickly feeling so much better, I see how bad it really is when it comes, and how much I suffer. And how that's not actually my fault and there is nothing I can do to stop it coming – it's something physiological in my brain. The triptan fixes that and I can function again. It's made me stop and think: dealing with a disease like this is hard, and thank goodness there are things that help."

I have seen a lot of this in myself and other migraine sufferers: we tend to downplay and disbelieve our own experience. Whether that's because once the pain is over, we can't perfectly remember how bad it was, or whether it's because there's no evidence for it that we can show someone else, I am not sure. But if, like Anita, you can believe yourself, you free yourself from so much of the suffering that comes from guilt. Because none of us should feel ashamed of being ill.

Amanda – not letting it stop you (from travelling)

Amanda didn't come to see me about migraines at all. She started therapy as a way to prepare herself for a big life change. At the age of 40, she was planning to leave her job as a market researcher and go travelling with her partner. He was a mechanic and was using his spare time to fit out a van for them to travel around Europe in. As the time came closer for them to leave and their plans began to take shape, Amanda found herself feeling increasingly anxious.

It was hard for us to pinpoint what exactly was making Amanda feel this anxiety. She was certainly pretty happy about swapping her job for a nomadic life, having put up with her share of the office politics and being ready for a change. She was a little worried about her dad, who'd been ill the previous year and was still recovering, but she did have a lot of faith that her twin sister would be able to keep an eye on him and keep her in the loop. She was a little worried about money, understandably, as travelling was potentially going to drain their savings – but, on reflection, she felt it was entirely worth it for this once-in-a-lifetime opportunity.

So, what was really bothering her? She was becoming increasingly vague, blaming "finding it difficult to get up" and "sometimes not really wanting to go outside very much". We looked into possible depression or underlying physical causes but didn't turn up much of significance.

Until I asked about periods. I always ask female clients about their periods at some point (not randomly, I hasten to add, I wait for the right moment, but it's nearly always a topic that gets them talking). Amanda had always had heavy periods and horrible period pains. Her sister somehow got away with periods that lasted four days and could be managed with a small box of tampons – she barely knew she was on. But Amanda's were a different animal. Their mother had died when they were 8 years old, and although their dad had told them about periods, he didn't have the personal experience angle. Amanda was left feeling like a freak for bleeding through her jeans and onto her bedding, and deeply ashamed of not being able to manage like her sister and other girls seemed to be able to.

I asked her if she ever got migraines with her periods and she said "No, but I did get this weird pulsing pain over my eyebrow. It made me feel quite sick and would last for days sometimes."

"You've just described a classic menstrual migraine, Amanda," I said.

"Have I? Is that what I've been having all this time?"

"I'd certainly recommend going and having a chat with your GP about it," I said. I can't diagnose these things, obviously, but it seemed pretty clear to me that she'd been suffering from migraines without realising that was what they were.

"I still get them – actually, it seems like I get one with every period just lately – and sometimes I even get them when I'm not on my period."

"And what are they like?"

"It's funny, I always wake up just fine, and then by the time I've had breakfast I know whether or not it's coming. I'm lying in bed, putting off getting upright, because I have this idea that it's being up and about that must bring them on. In the end, I get up because I think I ought to eat some breakfast, in case I feel horrible by mid morning and can't eat for the rest of the day."

"It stops you being able to eat, when you have this pain over your eyebrow?"

"Oh yes, I just can't face food at all then. And sometimes when I've forced myself, I've just been sick. It's a really peculiar kind of vomiting as well. It's not like when you've had something that's disagreed with you and you just feel much better after you've puked. It's like a really tough job to bring it up from the pit of your stomach, and then even when it's out, you still feel nauseated."

"That sounds horrible."

"I'm glad it doesn't happen every time, but I do worry about it happening when we're travelling. How will I manage then?"

I agreed that this was a very daunting prospect, and this led us to piece together where a lot of Amanda's anxiety was coming from. I urged her to go and have a chat with her GP about all of it, including the heaviness of her periods and the pain across one eyebrow, and see if they could help.

Unfortunately, the GP Amanda saw was dismissive, and sent her away with the suggestion that she pack some old towels to sleep on during her travels, and that perhaps seeing the grand sights of Europe would distract her from "annoying headaches". Amanda said she left the surgery feeling very small "and like I shouldn't be swapping my secure life here for a life on the road, and that doing so meant any problems were just all my fault."

"Do you think there's a chance the GP was a bit jealous of your travels?" I asked.

"Well, she did seem rather stressed out," Amanda conceded.

Sometimes we just catch GPs at the wrong moment, sometimes we ask them about something they've got no interest in or experience of and sometimes they just don't get it. Most of them are great people doing a tough job. I encouraged Amanda to try again, and ask for a different GP. It's worth remembering that you are always allowed to ask to see a different GP at your practice, and even a named one if there's someone you've had a good experience with before. This may mean waiting a little longer to see them, of course, but it can be so worth it. You can also ask if your surgery has any GPs who have a particular interest in migraine, menopause, perimenopausal issues or periods.

I was keen to hear from Amanda in our next session how her second appointment had gone. She had merely asked to see anyone except Dr Jealousy, and turned up for her appointment "to find this very young looking boy – my heart sank." However, this fresh-out-of-med-school young GP took Amanda very seriously and "he was surprisingly clued up on perimenopause". He listened to her experiences of heavy bleeding and painful migraines and sickness and took a full history from her. He asked her if she'd ever been on the contraceptive pill and she explained that she had tried it as a teen but found it had unacceptable side effects for her, so she'd never dallied with it again. He asked her if she'd reconsider it now, in either its combined or progesterone only form, and she said she'd go away and think about it. For the meantime, he prescribed her some codeine and told her to take it when the pain got bad, if OTC painkillers hadn't helped. He also assured her there were lots of options for managing both heavy periods and migraines, so he had hope they'd find something to help her. Just hearing those words helped Amanda a great deal. And finally, he ordered some blood tests to check how her iron levels were. He suspected that they might be depleted after years of heavy periods, a really not uncommon occurrence in menstruating women, and that low iron levels could even be contributing to the prevalence of her migraines.

Something Amanda and I worked very hard on together was being "migraine ready". Possibly because she'd spent years putting up with pain and not naming it as migraine, Amanda was unused to managing a migraine like it was a migraine. We constructed a plan. If she got up, had her breakfast, and then began to feel a migraine coming on, she would take some OTC painkillers. She would have plenty of these to hand at home, of course, but also she would ensure she always carried them to work and anywhere else she was going, so that she was never unable to medicate if she needed to. She also bought herself a large pair of dark glasses, and discovered that her reluctance to go outdoors was pretty much always paired with some sort of migraine pain. The dark glasses helped this not to feel as bad. The codeine really helped her if her first line treatment hadn't worked, and had the added bonus of making her feel so tired she needed to lie down. This meant that she often slept and recovered faster and was rarely sick anymore. She realised the vomiting had mainly occurred when she'd tried to fight through a migraine. In common with a lot of sufferers, she found that the stiller she kept, the better she felt and the sooner the migraine resolved.

Ultimately, she decided that hormonal contraceptives were not for her. She was able to try a different solution – mefenamic acid – to attempt to lighten her periods and make them less painful. Codeine continued to be useful to her, but she worried about taking it with her across Europe in the van. She was concerned about it being taken away from her at border control – it was possible to apply for and obtain the correct paperwork, but it was a risk she didn't want hanging over her.

This led her to ask for triptans instead, which she was able to try well ahead of the trip and figure out her dose.

We wound up our therapy a couple of weeks before she and her partner embarked on their trip. He'd built a cubby into the van for her to keep an epic supply of migraine pills, period supplies and a hot water bottle in: she felt as prepared as she could. She sent me a photo about three months later, of her sitting on the hood of the van, her dark glasses firmly on, with the Italian Riviera stretching out behind her.

"It's absolutely beautiful here, I'm really enjoying the view," she wrote, "but I couldn't be here if it weren't for the blackout blinds!"

I looked again at the photo and noticed the blackout blinds stretching across the van's windscreen. Amanda had packed them as part of her "migraine ready" kit, knowing that sometimes she'd just need to stop and lie in the back of the van in the dark. I was glad to hear that it wasn't stopping her from doing at least some of the travelling she had so wanted to do.

Nicole – managing nausea

When Nicole first got in touch with me, she said that she wanted to talk through "ageing". I pictured an older lady, perhaps, coming to work through loss of mobility or identity. I was quite surprised to meet Nicole for the first time and be faced with a tall, athletic woman in her mid-40s. She carried herself very confidently until she got settled into a chair, and then she crumpled and began to cry.

"I'm so sorry," she sobbed into a tissue, "I just don't know who I am this past year...I used to be full of energy and laugh a lot...and now I watch my wife chase our kids around the park and I'm too tired to join in. I used to run several times a week – now if I try I end up with a migraine most times, and it's just not worth the risk. My hair's falling out and my skin feels shrivelled and...I went to my GP and he said there was no way it was menopause, I'm too young. So I'm left wondering why I feel like such an old lady and if my life is actually over!"

I explained to Nicole that, at 46 years of age, she was actually at the prime age for perimenopause, and how her GP seemed to have that muddled with menopause itself. She'd actually done a fair bit of reading around it and seen Davina McCall's documentary, so she wasn't surprised to hear that and found it validating – it's just that the word of a GP can seem to be the "gold standard" and the thing we should really trust. The reality is that some GPs have had no training at all in perimenopause and menopause issues or are working on outdated or incomplete information.

Nicole told me how her periods had actually been quite manageable up until the past year, when suddenly her regular cycle had become unpredictable. Sometimes she'd been caught out when a period arrived just two weeks after the last one, and other times she was a whole month late and then had what she described as a "monster period" – much heavier than she was used to, and with debilitating cramps that saw her taking days off work and having to curl up with a hot water bottle.

She had also regularly experienced migraines – perhaps 4-6 a year – since she was a teenager, but hadn't thought they were connected with her periods as they always seemed to come in the middle of her cycle, and not around the time of her bleed. She would always know when they were coming as she would see zigzag patterns at the edges of her vision, and then have a slightly "swimmy" feeling for an hour or two before the pain arrived, always on one side of her head, just over her brow and digging into the temple. We talked about how this could well be migraine with aura, which does seem to be associated with rises in oestrogen (whereas migraine without aura is more associated with oestrogen dips). We explored the theory that perhaps her migraines had always arrived in the middle of her cycle because that was when she was ovulating, and her oestrogen was highest.

It made sense that, since her periods had gone awry, her migraines had increased too. Exercise certainly seemed to be a trigger for them but, as Nicole noted, not always, and perhaps this meant she was most vulnerable when her oestrogen was surging. The only thing was, there was no way to know when the surges would be, since perimenopause was putting everything in flux. "Unless I could have a blood test every single day, I'm not going to know until I see those zigzags that I have a migraine coming," she said.

This made being a parent to twin five year olds and a three year old more demanding than it already was. When the kids were babies, Nicole had enjoyed being the one who nurtured her wife after she'd given birth, and took up the 3am nappies and feeds. Nowadays she often had to retreat to bed – or, more frequently, the bathroom so she could throw up – while her wife tried to juggle the three under-fives.

Nicole's migraines tended to make her very sick and for her this was more incapacitating than the pain. "I can smile through the pain somewhat," she told me, "but I can't hide having to throw up on the school run." Another mum had tried to make her feel better by commiserating with the words "Rough night, was it? We've all had those!" It only had the effect of making Nicole feel sure all the other parents were wondering if she was an alcoholic.

It also put stress on her marriage. Her wife was understandably feeling the strain of doing most of the childcare and never knowing whether Nicole would be there or not. But her wife also noticed that Nicole was becoming increasingly anxious about going out anywhere, in case an attack came on and she had to throw up in public, and this seemed like a huge pivot from the outgoing woman she married. "Sadie is ten years younger than me and I just feel myself ageing super fast ahead of her," Nicole explained, "which is not helped by my libido being in the toilet either." Another common symptom of perimenopause.

Between me suggesting it and her wife pleading with her to do it, Nicole booked another visit to the GP. I felt sure that, armed with a bit more education about migraines with aura and perimenopause, Nicole would be able to get what she needed from the appointment. I was a bit surprised when she came back the following week to tell me she'd been prescribed antidepressants.

"I know, I found it confusing at first too, when the GP suggested it. I did explain about my symptoms and why I thought it was all perimenopause-related, but he really clocked onto my anxiety around going out and my inability to go running, which he said showed I might be depressed. He felt very strongly I should try this first, and frightened me with a bunch of stats around HRT and cancer that I didn't really take in."

"Is there a family history of cancer that he might have needed to be concerned about?" I asked.

"No...no, nothing like that. He just emphasised the link between HRT and cancer risks."

It's not uncommon for GPs to prescribe antidepressants for perimenopausal symptoms, since many of them can look like depression, and anxiety can really ramp up at this life stage. They do tend to help with mood swings and PMS. However, I knew they wouldn't do anything for Nicole's migraines or nausea, both of which had been ignored, and which seemed to me to be causing her difficulties with going out and enjoying things as she used to.

It's also not uncommon for GPs to hang onto old information about HRT. A very long time ago, HRT was made of horse wee. Nowadays, it is bio-identical and derived from the humble yam[xiv]. Also a long time ago, there was a study done about HRT and cancer risk that claimed women were at high risk if they took HRT[xv]. The study was flawed in a number of ways and has since been discredited, but its legacy remains lodged in the minds of doctors (and many patients).

Nowadays there is evidence that the increased risk of breast cancer is low[xvi] – though extra care needs to be taken for women who have a family history of breast cancer or who have a cancer history themselves. A GP should refer such women to a specialist to work out what HRT they can have, if any, in their particular circumstances. For everyone else, the slightly elevated risk of breast and ovarian cancer is often considered acceptable if the benefits outweigh them. Unfortunately, there isn't much evidence that HRT helps prevent perimenopausal migraines, but there's a lot of evidence that it can help with other troubling perimenopause symptoms, like loss of libido, thinning hair and skin, and vaginal dryness[xvii].

Nicole decided to give the antidepressants a trial and see how she felt. It was somewhat difficult to judge as she experienced a lot of migraine with vomiting during this time and was not convinced she kept much of the medication in her system some days, but after a month she was sure she wasn't deriving any benefit. She couldn't face going back to her GP, and asking to see a third different doctor, so she decided to visit an online menopause clinic. She took care to select a reputable one with highly respectable credentials and solid reviews. Of course, it cost her a fee, but she decided to try it anyway.

I was eager to hear about her experience in our next session. The thing that struck her the most was that, although it was an online session, she'd been given a whole hour to discuss her symptoms with a doctor, who really listened and checked she'd understood how things were affecting Nicole. The doctor also ran through some possible treatment options and explained clearly the risks and possible benefits of HRT, so that Nicole could make an informed decision. In fact, she didn't even make her decision on the spot, as there was no pressure, and she took the time to go away and discuss it all with Sadie. Then she got back to the doctor and said she would like to try HRT, which would hopefully help with her libido and fatigue. The doctor was optimistic that it may help with the migraines too, but advised Nicole to return to her GP if she still needed help with that side of things. She also cautioned Nicole not to come off her antidepressants suddenly, and to ensure she sought her GP's advice about stepping down slowly to avoid unpleasant side effects.

The HRT prescription was with Nicole within a few days and she got started. After a couple of weeks, she reported feeling a bit more energetic and had noticed her hair and skin felt more like they used to. These benefits alone gave her some hope, and perhaps the boost she needed to return to her GP and talk further about the migraines. She certainly didn't feel like having much sex, but she reasoned that "no one feels sexy when they're nauseated or their head is on fire."

She ended up seeing a locum GP who turned out to be a migraine sufferer herself. She warned Nicole that, while migraines are well known as being difficult to treat, perimenopausal migraines are the most difficult subtype to treat. She was trying to adjust Nicole's expectations as she prescribed a triptan and some anti-nausea medication. She didn't want to promise the Earth – after all, we can't cure migraine, and the most Nicole might realistically be able to hope for was a reduction in the number of migraines she had.

However, the triptans did really work for Nicole. She had been instructed to take a triptan *not* at the start of her aura, but immediately as the pain arrived. She always knew when it was coming because of the aura symptoms, and would be ready with her triptan as soon as the pain began. She found that if she took the triptan at the point of pain onset, the pain would be gone completely within about twenty minutes. Plus, it never took a real hold, so she never felt dreadfully sick.

The doctor had told her that she could take as many as ten triptans per month, and this easily covered her migraine days. For a couple of months she was absolutely migraine free and felt as close to her old self again as she thought possible. And she did get her sex drive back: it was still challenging to find time for sex, with three children running around and taking up most of her and Sadie's energy, "but at least the desire is there," she smiled, with no small degree of relief.

Nicole put her focus on other things in therapy, now that her migraine and perimenopause issues felt like they were under control. It was perhaps three months later when she had to cancel a session because a migraine had brought her to a standstill. We rearranged the session for when she was feeling better and she explained, quite tearfully, that the triptan hadn't worked that time. She'd taken it as usual, just as soon as the pain came on, but after watching the clock for an hour she felt worse, not better, and she had begun to feel sick. She remembered her anti nausea medication, which she took and found really helped take the edge off that side of things. But the pain knocked her out for a couple of days.

Her doctor had explained that if a triptan gives you some relief, but then the pain returns within two hours, she could take a second triptan. However, she should not take a second one if the first one hadn't worked at all or had given at least two hours of pain relief. What we figured out as the weeks rolled on was that most of the time, her triptan was a "magic bullet". Some of the time, it just gave her a few hours of relief. Some of the time, it did nothing at all. In those cases, she took her anti-nausea meds, and tried her best to "smile through the pain". If she couldn't, she had to go to bed.

One thing she did notice was that she felt less anxious once she had a medication plan for her migraines, and this was something I really identified with. OK, the triptans might not work perfectly all the time, but the fact of having them and knowing what to expect from them meant Nicole understood what she could do and what she might be dealing with. The anti-nausea medication was a massive help with going out and about, too, as it meant she no longer worried about throwing up in public. She learned some relaxation exercises for the times when the pain floored her, so that at least she didn't add any unnecessary physical tension into the mix. And while she never got back to her running, she did enjoy chasing her kids around the park again and going on long walks.

Danielle – when it's trauma related

Danielle had been my client for a couple of years before we even discussed migraine. She'd first come to see me at the age of 36, just as her daughter was forging her own path into independence, and Danielle finally felt she had enough time and energy to seek professional help with some things she'd been managing alone for a while.

Danielle was a survivor of child sex abuse (CSA) and we'd worked for about two years on what she remembered about her experiences, how she had got through it at the time and how it was impacting her now. She had been sexually abused for much of her childhood by her dad and brother, and occasionally by an uncle as well. Her main way of coping with the sexual encounters they forced on her was to "vanish" into her imagination. She had constructed an entire universe of magical characters in her mind who populated fantastical landscapes and got into scrapes and adventures. She cast herself as the heroine of this fantasy world, where she had special powers to heal other creatures.

At school she had been praised for some of the stories she wrote, as of course she always had one at her fingertips from her fantasy land, and other kids loved playing with her because she dreamt up such involving games full of fairies and dragons. However, it also got her into trouble, when she was found to be disappearing into her own world instead of joining in with some class activity. She didn't realise at the time, but this usually happened when they were asked to do something that reminded her of closeness or relationships (PSHE was a particularly tricky topic) because naturally she had some really conflicted feelings about those that she couldn't process. No one picked up on this link, nor did the GP question the number of UTIs she suffered from. Even several years later, when she wrote and performed a piece for GCSE Drama all about CSA, no one asked her if it was personal. Her Drama teacher just gave her an outstanding grade for the authenticity of her acting.

Danielle never thought directly to herself that she must tell someone what was going on, because like a lot of CSA survivors, she assumed this was probably happening to everyone. It's hard to know any different when you are a child. She had this vague hope that someone would figure out she wasn't OK and perhaps teach her some secret to putting up with it. She also imagined there was a worldwide implicit agreement that although everyone went through this, no one talked about it. And then she kept disappearing into her imagination to cope and get some respite.

Danielle had a particularly tough time when she left home. She fell into an abusive relationship with a man who treated her in much the same way as the male members of her family had. However, he was physically violent towards her in a way they hadn't been, and when she ended up in A&E having stitches in her face, an astute nurse found an opportunity to ask her about what was really going on. The police were called and Danielle's partner was charged with assault. On the same night, an A&E doctor gave her the news that she was 6 weeks pregnant, and she was thrown into chaos. It was when an on call social worker suggested she return home to her dad for some safety and respite that she told everything, and made allegations about her dad, brother and uncle.

While she was supported to go through the police interview and give evidence against her family, the case never made it to court. As in so many CSA cases, it all fell down on lack of forensic evidence. Danielle was left to fend for herself, as a single mother, feeling terrified of repercussions from all of her abusers.

Thankfully, she was granted social housing in a different area of the country from where her abusers were, and she changed her name and didn't tell anyone in her new neighbourhood where she'd come from or, indeed, much about herself at all. She ended up liking her new neighbourhood a lot, as it was full of young families and was a fresh start. She felt like she had a mission to look after her new baby girl and keep them both safe. A friendly neighbour put her onto a job working part time in an accountancy office, where she answered phones and generated invoices and organised meetings. Between her office hours and taking care of a little one, she barely had time to slip into her fantasy world anymore – but then, she didn't need it so much these days. Perhaps only as she slipped into bed at night, tired, but still feeling those old fears about going to sleep. Nighttime had never been a safe time in her old life.

By the time she came to see me, she was ready to start looking at some of the things that were still causing her pain: the nighttime panic came high up the list, but there was also the misplaced blame (common among CSA survivors), the anger about the lack of justice, the repeat trauma as she found she was "only attracted to bullies" and got into damaging relationships, and the loss of any family connection or identity. As well as being her abusers, her family had been her earliest caregivers, and not all her memories of them were bad ones. This kind of mixed bag can be really hard to carry.

Building trust, helping Danielle spot relational patterns, dissolving misplaced blame and shame and processing anger and loss takes time, and we kept at our work in those first couple of years. Danielle was a thinker: she reflected and journaled a lot between sessions and often shared these insights with me. I admired her tenacity and felt she was making good progress.

She had said it was tough being in therapy, and that sometimes she felt forgetful or a bit absent in other areas of her life because she was processing so many thoughts. She reported feeling hot and cold, and sometimes waking up in the night soaked through with sweat – which she put down to her common nightmares.

But then she began to complain of migraines. I wasn't surprised to hear that they often came on after a heavy therapy session, or when she'd been thinking about the abuse a lot, or after particularly disturbing nightmares. But then they began happening whenever she did something fairly demanding, like concentrating hard to take minutes in an hour-long meeting at work, or attending a talk at the local library about a topic she was interested in, but which required that she take in a lot of new information.

"I get this feeling of my head being very full," she said, "and then pain comes along with it, always down one side. It can last for hours." She began trying every OTC remedy she could think of to abate the pain: paracetamol and ibuprofen were "a waste of time", hayfever tablets "did literally nothing" (she had read online they helped some people), codeine made her feel dizzy and sick, and complementary medicines like tiger balm and cool packs "just didn't do a thing." She blamed herself for getting "so stressed about things" but actually I saw her as a woman who was gradually becoming more comfortable with managing difficult emotions and the legacy of her past. I gently brought up the other symptoms she'd told me about and suggested that there might be a link with the perimenopause. At 38, she was horrified, but I explained that with the perimenopause starting probably ten years before going through menopause itself, she wasn't far ahead of the curve – and there is evidence to suggest trauma survivors may go through menopause sooner. She booked herself in with the GP for a chat.

"Do you think the GP will just look at my records though and say that of course I have migraines, I've been through some shit?"

I knew she was really worried about going to this appointment and not being believed, never mind being offered any help.

"GPs are so busy they usually don't have time to read much of your notes ahead of seeing you," I said. "If they've read the reason you gave for booking the appointment, then they're as prepared as they can be sometimes."

As it turned out, this GP did not read Danielle's full history, and the appointment ran so much the better for it. She listened to Danielle's concerns about night sweats, brain fog and migraines and nodded in agreement when Danielle mentioned the perimenopause. She suggested some HRT but also sent

Danielle away with a pack of triptans to try, urging her to come back for another check in after a month.

"I felt so relieved that she took me seriously," Danielle told me later, "but I still felt the need to tell her I was having therapy too, so she didn't think I was expecting tablets to fix it all."

"And Danielle, even if she had known about your history, and you were not in therapy, you're still in pain and you still deserve treatment," I said.

I think this is true no matter what the cause of our migraines. We can't expect any course of treatment to guarantee that we won't feel any more pain, but we can expect to have a shot at treatment – whether that's preventative meds, painkillers, triptans, anti-nausea pills and whether or not that's combined with our own efforts to help ourselves. Obviously if we can help ourselves we tend to get more benefit, rather than simply relying on medication to do the legwork, but I don't think it would ever be fair to withhold migraine treatment from someone because they weren't proactively dealing with their sources of stress. It's amazing how much a reduction in physical pain can free up bandwidth for a person to better manage their emotional pain, too.

Over the next few months it became apparent that the HRT was working to lift Danielle's brain fog and night sweats pretty effectively. She felt more alert but continued to get that "full head" feeling which would usually lead to a migraine. The triptan she tried had no impact, so she did return to her GP and tried a different one. That didn't work for her, either. There are seven different kinds of triptans but once Danielle got onto number 4 without success, she gave up. Her doctor put her on Amitriptyline and that did, after about a month, reduce the number of migraines by about a third. She managed to be astonishingly glass-half-full about it, remarking that she was glad it hadn't happened while her daughter was younger, when she would have been unable to take care of her sometimes, and that she was grateful her employer (where she'd stayed for years by this point) was so understanding and flexible.

She also didn't give up on finding things to relieve the migraines. She tried, it seemed to me, a different remedy each week almost, reporting on how they had or hadn't worked in our sessions.

"Well this week it's been fish!" she said to me one week.

"I'm sorry, fish?" I checked.

"Yep! I read online that a lack of omega 3 fatty acids can cause migraines, so I've tried to eat some mackerel or tuna every day."

"And how's that going?"

"Well, I've had two migraines and I'm absolutely sick of fish," she confessed.

The only thing she did have some success with was Botox. This works by temporarily blocking some of the pain signals carried by neurotransmitters. However, at at least £500 for a treatment, which would wear off after twelve weeks, this wasn't something she could keep up easily. She coped by eking out the time between treatments as much as possible, so that she had closer to two treatments a year than four.

We also learned in therapy how to spot that "full head" feeling. Danielle would let me know if she felt it coming on, or I would ask if I saw her frowning or rubbing the side of her head or yawning. If we could spot the overwhelm, we would stop talking and I would direct her through a breathing exercise. This helped us to pace the session more slowly and perhaps we prevented some of her attacks that way. She tried to use this technique outside sessions too, but admitted it was often too hard to give up speed and competence for slowness and self care. She didn't want to draw attention to her struggles, and would usually choose keeping it all in her head rather than showing that anything was wrong. I say she would choose, but this was such an old and deeply rooted pattern from her early life that I think it was more of an instinct. In therapy, she learned that nothing bad happened if she stopped the work and breathed and slowed down. Our continuing work was about gradually risking that outside the therapy room, and hoping to see fewer and fewer migraines as well.

Something I know about working with trauma is that you often don't do it once. Trauma can come back up for reevaluation at any stage of your life, but perhaps particularly during a life stage transition or other big change. This was certainly something Danielle identified with.

"I used to feel like I dealt with a lot of my trauma when I moved away from home and started over, and then when I became a mum and gave my girl a very different experience of childhood – that really healed some things for me," she reflected. "I guess my coming into therapy with you when I did was no coincidence. Not only did I have a bit more time on my own to think, but I was also gearing up to this big change with my hormones and this new stage of life."

I think she got it spot on. Sometimes when something big happens in the here and now, it shuffles the deck beneath us and brings old stuff to the surface for a bit more processing. This doesn't mean you didn't do the processing "right" or thoroughly enough the first time around. It just means that different bits of the processing become relevant as time moves on and things change in our lives.

Summary

My work with all my clients is varied and complex. The above are just a glimpse into some of what might go on in therapy relating to perimenopausal migraines which, of course, are integrated into other issues in our lives. While every client is different and my work with each will not be the same, there are some common threads that come up, which you may have picked up on. These are:

- **Recognising that it's migraine.** So many people talk about "annoying headaches" and "head pain" and

"niggles" when what they mean is migraine. Migraine is a one sided, pulsating or thumping intermittent pain that can usually be located over the eyebrow, the temple and sometimes all the way into the neck and jaw in one direction and up to the scalp in the other. The distinction is crucial because treatment of a headache is very different to the treatment options for migraine. Often neglecting to call a migraine what it is is about our anxiety not to "cause a fuss" or a mistrust in our own experience.
- **Feeling guilty.** Whether we're missing work or crucial milestones in our children's lives, flaking on friends or having to scale back the help we offer others, the guilt that comes with migraine (and any chronic illness) is real. Focus on what you can do, and work towards understanding why you couldn't do more.
- **Not being listened to the first time.** Or sometimes the second, third or fourth time, unfortunately. Don't give up. You will find a good GP or menopause or migraine specialist. It can help to show up at appointment with your migraine diary (see next chapter) and a list of symptoms and/or questions you want to raise. This can take some of the stress out of explaining it all on the fly – especially if your appointment falls on a migraine day.
- **Accepting that it probably won't be a 100% solution.** Some people do get cured from migraine. But most often, this challenging condition can be managed and worked with, rather than cured. Adjust your own expectations and find a doctor who is on the same page.
- **Migraine involves loss.** You are going to miss out sometimes. You might lose some friends. You might lose opportunities. You'll doubtless lose money and sleep. Some people even lose partners or jobs. You're allowed to be sad about all that loss. But try not to let it swamp you. You can still do things and you will feel better.

Ways I've managed perimenopausal migraines

Here is a comprehensive list of the things I did to help me manage my perimenopausal migraines. I've split them into two broad categories: good things (things I would happily recommend to others) and bad things (please don't try these at home. I include them so that you don't have to try them).

Of course, what works for one person doesn't necessarily work for another. And none of these are 100% solutions, not even close. But sometimes the best we can do is the things that help by 5% or 10%, and those things are worth having.

Always check with a doctor before you try anything you're unsure about. Ideally, this section gives you some ideas for treatment that you can take to a health provider and use to talk about what might be right for you. What follows is not medical advice, merely the sharing of one person's individual experience.

Part of managing migraines is accepting that there is no reliable cure for them. There is much hope, but not all migraines can be taken away or even dampened down. We are going to lose some of our lives to them. I do suspect that migraines *could* actually be fail-safe cured if we were given large enough doses of morphine or something, but that might well solve one problem while opening up a whole bunch of others. And opiate addiction is more life limiting than migraines are.

Having said that, I'm going to start by talking about painkillers...

Ways I've managed (good)

Painkillers

It is difficult to overstate how much painkillers have helped me on this journey through perimenopausal migraine. I was never one of those people who considered their body too precious to put a paracetamol in it, but this has swayed me further towards having faith in how drugs work.

It seems to be the case that taking a painkiller early in a migraine episode ups your chances of aborting the thing before it takes hold, or at least dampening the pain for a while or the speed at which the attack comes on. It is by no means a guarantee. Plenty of times I have taken something at the first pain (because I don't get an aura, pain is my first sign) and ended up with a raging migraine anyway. But I feel sure I have prevented a lot of suffering by simply getting an aspirin into myself pronto.

The reason to be cautious about painkillers is that by taking too many of any of them, including the simple ones like paracetamol and ibuprofen, you can cause something called a Medication Overuse Headache. The guidance is not to take simple painkillers for more than 15 days in the month, and not to take combination painkillers (like ibuprofen and codeine together) for more than 10. It doesn't specify whether that means 15 days of taking one dose of ibuprofen per day is the threshold, or whether you can take the maximum cocktail of painkillers you're allowed (usually 4 daily doses of one thing, spaced at least 4 hours apart) and still be safe from MOH, but hey. You'll know you have MOH if you have a dull, constant headache that's pesky but not as violent as a migraine. Just for funsies, you'll continue to get migraines inbetween the MOHs. But basically, in trying your best to treat your horrible migraines, you can end up giving yourself more head pain, which just doesn't seem fair at all.

Essentially MOH is caused by drug withdrawal. Previously I always assumed the kinds of drugs that caused withdrawal symptoms were the big ones like heroin, so I thought I would never have to worry about an innocent little paracetamol. But all drugs are drugs and, if they're effective, then they're also going to have downsides.

I have read migraine books about treating migraine with peppermint oil and positive thoughts and without exception left them scathing online reviews. I cannot advocate for the drug-free approach. Sorry, the drugs have just been too sodding helpful too much of the time (though not all the time – the drugs have got some progress to make). But I do urge treating any drugs you use with the utmost respect.

Keep a migraine diary that includes what you took and when, and whether it helped. It will help you know exactly how much and how often you are using which painkillers, and you can adhere to the guidelines to avoid MOH. If in any doubt, hand your migraine diary to a trusted person, who will add up what you've had and how often (you are not living your best maths life when migraining), and hopefully bring you a big glass of water and the drug of your choice. If still in any doubt, hand your migraine diary to your GP, and they will soon tell you if you're within acceptable parameters or not.

There is a strong case for not using codeine at all in the treatment of migraine. It is known to be more likely to cause MOH (hence the 10 day, rather than 15 day limit) and it is also known to be potentially addictive in a way that ibuprofen/paracetamol/aspirin isn't. These seem like excellent reasons to steer clear of it and if that's what you decide to do, that seems entirely sensible.

Two things kept me using it: it was the thing that worked best for a long time, and it gave me a lovely feeling of calm. One of the things that bothers me a lot about migraine (aside from the sickening pain, sensitivity to sound and light, the general hell...) is the anxiety that comes with it. My aching head can send my brain off in a dozen directions urgently, just at the very time when it would be most useful to slow my roll. The mellow buzz of codeine slows me by a few degrees and gives me a reassuring sense of it really being OK to relax. Ideally, I'd learn to achieve that without any codeine. And I have put work into that, believe me, and I can get a long way with that when I am well. But when I am migraining, it is almost inaccessible. Something about pain sets off a whole body and brain emergency alarm in my system, and codeine just comes along and wraps a blanket around it and muffles it quite a lot.

One of the reasons I think this is OK is that I never ever want to take codeine when I am well. It is utterly at odds with my pain-free self, who is excited about getting All The Things done, and quite happy to bound along at a merry old speed. Without pain in the equation, my brain running fast feels productive and exhilarating and helpful, plus I have learned to slow it if it would be useful to dial down the puppy (in most therapy sessions, for example). This may be naïve of me, but I feel this means I am unlikely to be at risk of becoming addicted. I suppose the evidence is that I have used it for almost a decade without becoming an addict.

However, I think it's telling that it doesn't work as well on me as it used to. In the early years, I would take it (30mg on its own when I had that initial prescription, but mainly in the form of over-the-counter (OTC) 12mg codeine combined with paracetamol or ibuprofen) for my migraine and it would lift the whole thing away quickly and lastingly. I rarely needed more than one dose per day.

Perhaps two or three years in, I started to find it wore off, rather than erasing the migraine for the whole day at a time. I never exceeded the guidelines on the packet, but sometimes I needed to take a dose eight hours after the first, sometimes as soon as four hours after.

And not so long after that, while it still helped, it didn't always take a migraine away. It stopped being my guaranteed method of aborting migraine. It's still that way for me. I will take my simple painkiller and then, if that does nothing, and I haven't deemed this a triptan day, then I will take the combined codeine and paracetamol (if my initial pick was ibuprofen or aspirin) or codeine and ibuprofen (if my initial pick was paracetamol). It will almost always take the pain down a notch. Sometimes several. And sometimes it gets rid of it completely. But it feels much more pot luck these days.

This could be a sign that I have a higher tolerance for codeine owing to having used it regularly. I have never exceeded the limits of 10 days per month. I have also never exceeded the limits either set by a doctor or stated on the back of the packet. And yet my body still seems to have got used to it, and where it once said "Yippee!" when I took it, it now sometimes says "Meh."

That's obviously not great. What if I need codeine at some future date because of some other kind of pain? But then, I figure migraine is almost the worst pain I have ever experienced (I reserve the top spot for induced labour pain). I broke my toe during the pandemic and didn't want to go to A&E, so I didn't. The pain was pretty background compared to a migraine, in all honesty. So, although I don't know what my pain relief needs are going to be in the future, I don't regret using codeine to relieve migraines because for a significant period it really helped me to get on with my life.

I do accept that it isn't a good long term solution. I really think it needs to be prescribed and/or self administered with the utmost of care. Definitely tell someone you're taking it, preferably a medical professional. And write it all in your migraine diary, so you can keep a check on how much you're taking and when. Write it as you take it, because your migraine will ensure your memory is unreliable. And if you are ever tempted to take it when you're well, or you think you're taking more than you should, get help.

Triptans

Triptans are now considered the best migraine treatment we have available[xviii]. There is a promising new family of drugs, known as gepants, which have just become available recently on the NHS, which may be even more effective. But, for a while now, triptans have been the gold standard.

They are not painkillers: rather they work by changing the way blood flows through your brain, and influencing how pain signals are interpreted by mimicking serotonin (a neurotransmitter we have naturally in our brains that plays a role in managing pain, among other things).

It is worth knowing that there are several different triptans. The first one I tried didn't help me, but the second one did. It is not a magic bullet: taking a triptan buys me about six to eight hours "off". The migraine usually comes back after that window. And it can take up to two hours for the triptan to take effect in the first place. But once it kicks in, it often erases all traces of the migraine for a blissful spell of time. This is valuable if you have special occasion or a really important thing to do that requires you to be migraine-free.

They have limitations. I was told not to take more than six per month (indeed, I can only get six prescribed per month) although general guidance seems to be an upper limit of ten per month[xix]. There is also guidance to suggest it is not a good idea to take a triptan more than two or three times per week. This is because of the risks of Medication Overuse Headache, which can also occur with triptans even though they are not painkillers.

If you are getting chronic migraine (more than fifteen migraine days per month) as I was for some time, clearly triptans are not going to take it all away. But they will buy you a break. That, combined with other painkillers and trying to manage your triggers (see below) will sometimes help.

Knowing about triggers

I think of the hormonal punk rockery causing my migraines as a bonfire: it is there all the time, at certain times built higher than others, and sometimes it will spontaneously catch fire and burn my head down. Other times, the bonfire is there but it is waiting for a spark – or a trigger – to actually start a blaze. The triggers don't cause the migraine, in that they would be harmless if the bonfire weren't there.

One of my triggers is sunlight. If my bonfire is already built, and I go out on a sunny day without dark glasses, I will quickly have a migraine. It's a strong trigger for me, meaning that it almost always causes a migraine. If the bonfire is smaller (hormones a bit more settled that day) maybe sunlight triggers a less catastrophic headache, easily assuaged by a couple of paracetamol. If the bonfire is bigger (hormones doing all kinds of crazy stuff in the background) I could trigger a worse and longer lasting attack.

My list of triggers is long and range from the common ones you'd easily guess to the completely ridiculous. As well as sunlight, my triggers are: being too hot, not getting enough sleep, concentrating too hard, being dehydrated, adrenaline, stress, anxiety, hunger, eye strain, doing too much exercise, having another illness like a cold or fever, repetitive noise at certain frequencies (power tools are especially bad), two competing verbal inputs (trying to listen to a conversation while a podcast is playing, for example), electric lights if they shine in my eyes at all (my house is full of small lamps with lampshades), a car coming towards me at the wrong angle at night so its headlights shine in my eyes, doing something new or out of routine and travelling.

Once a migraine is blazing, almost anything can make it worse. Any sounds, any light source. I am lucky that smells don't seem to trigger me or make me worse (except it's often not fun to smell food of any kind when you're nauseated). That's not the case for all migraine sufferers though, and those folk have my sympathy. Those people can walk into a room where someone is wearing the wrong kind of perfume and have a migraine instantly.

Once you know what triggers you (and what doesn't) you can, to an extent, work with those things. I can't avoid sunlight (unless I want to adopt a vampire lifestyle) but I do own several pairs of sunglasses so I always have a pair to hand. Make life easier for yourself and have a pair in your bag, a pair in the car, a pair by the back door for when you "just" want to nip into the garden and then regret it instantly as the sunlight shoves a pointy dagger into your eye.

For me, dark glasses work. For some people, a coloured filter is better, like blue tinted or yellow tinted glasses. Whatever makes you feel more comfortable. And if you need them on in a brightly lit or sunny room, or just an averagely lit room, put them on. Some people will think you're being a wannabe rock star dick. Those people do not have migraines.

What about when you can't avoid a trigger? Like your day is stressful for reasons beyond your control, or you really have to concentrate very hard on something? That's where you do your best not to add any other triggers into the mix. If you can stay extra hydrated, eat well, take a break or nap, get some peace and quiet and dim the lights, maybe it won't be too bad. It'll definitely be better than dealing with multiple triggers, anyway.

And what about when you really want to do something that triggers you? Like staying up past 10pm, for example. Most times, if I dare have so much of a life that I am not in my bed by 10pm, a migraine will descend around half past ten, eleven latest. And you needn't think, as I did optimistically several times, that I can just sleep that off. It will still be ramming into my temple at 2am, until I finally give up and take something for it, and try to salvage some sleep.

But sometimes I choose to be up past 10pm anyway. Am I going to turn down every social occasion that ends past that time? No. Sometimes I decide the price of a migraine is one I'm willing to pay in order not to miss being at that party or gig or seeing that friend. I will just be extra prepared the next day for the migraine.

If I were to keep on top of all my triggers all of the time, that would be my full time job. I still trip up with them regularly, because it is hard to stay out of sunlight while simultaneously staying the right temperature, sleeping at the right times, drinking three pints of water, eating to schedule, combating stress, avoiding power tools and staying calm. That's a lot of plates to spin and I can't always do it.

So don't expect yourself to manage your triggers perfectly even if you know what all of them are. Think in terms of working with them as best you can and developing good habits that help with that. But let yourself off if you accidentally or purposefully let a plate drop.

Friends

I lucked out with my friends. Not one of them has dropped me for cancelling on them *yet again* because I have a migraine. Perhaps it has to do with being honest about it. I used to often say I "just can't make it" or apologise but not give a reason for cancelling. There was definitely some shame on my part for being ill (again) but also a lack of trust that the other person would understand. Usually people really *do* understand. Estimates suggest around 10 million adults in the UK experience migraine[xx], so your chances are good that they've either had one or they love someone who suffers. And if someone drops you because you had a migraine, they're not the kind of dickhead you need in your life.

My best friend, who I have known since our secondary school days, is brilliant. In much the same way that when we were 14 she let me blather on about how much I loved New Kids on the Block, she seems OK with hearing all about my migraines. She even asks about them. And where I am conscious with most other people not to go on and on about it, I do let myself tell her the truth. Her, and my husband. I recommend having a couple of people you really do tell it like it is to.

The reason for this is that saying things out loud, and feeling safe enough not to filter, has a magical effect. I witness it in therapy all the time. It doesn't lead to wallowing in self pity (and most of us don't want pity from the other person either) – quite the opposite. Being able to say it all aloud, to someone who has empathy for us, allows us to face it how it is – and however bad it is. It takes some clever brain processing to take the thoughts and feelings residing in our heads and turn them into words and sentences that someone else can understand, and a bonus side product of that processing is acceptance. A kind of ah-ha, this is what I mean. This is how things are. And once we can grasp that, however far from ideal it is, we can begin to cope with it.

There is something to be said for connecting with others who are going through something similar. That might not be a friend or indeed anyone you know, but perhaps an online community of some kind. I am fortunate to have a friend, Marie, who's been a bit of a chronic illness partner for me, mostly via email. I worked with her twenty years ago, before migraine was much of a thing for me, and we've stayed in touch mainly via email ever since. We used to live a long distance from each other, so we got into the habit of emailing back and forth. Nowadays, we live in easy meeting distance, but we still carry on the majority of our friendship via email. I'm sure that both of us having been English teachers once has much to do with this, but it also lends space to the dynamic. We often open and/or close our emails to each other with some variation on: "Don't feel pressured to respond until you're having a good day and have time."

Marie doesn't have migraine. She has another chronic illness that means she's dealing with a lot of fatigue and brain fog, among other things. There's definitely enough crossover that she gets all my challenges (and I hope I get hers well enough too). I never have to explain to Marie. She already knows.

This has been a boon for all sorts of reasons. She's given me tips for coping (like "look at what you've managed to do each day, not what you didn't manage") and generously shared her own experiences, good and bad. She's sometimes gently admonished me ("Of course you shouldn't have pushed yourself to do x in the middle of a migraine! But I know I have done the same!") and often validated me ("You were so right to curl up in bed/take your medication/not expect so much of yourself"). She's also super funny and has made me laugh about migraine, pain and fatigue. It's a dark humour, admittedly, but it does help to laugh about it.

Marie is one of those friends you can arrange to go out with and know that you will manage no matter what your migraine is throwing at you. I can cancel on her, knowing she will understand. I can go home early if I need to, and she won't take it personally. One day, shortly after things opened up again as the worst of the Covid lockdown eased, I arranged to meet Marie in a cafe in Cambridge. I was on day three of a migraine and feeling spectacularly bad, but I knew she would get it if my words were garbled and I wasn't great company. It is just always a comfort to be in her company, so off I went.

We found ourselves sat in quite a busy cafe, mid morning, me with my booming head and sicky feeling, and her dealing with her own chronic illness symptoms. A masked waitress came up to take our order. Before the waitress could get through her opening spiel, Marie let her know:

"We're both quite unwell today."

Just like that: no shame or apology. The waitress took a step back from us.

"It's OK – migraine and chronic fatigue type stuff – not Covid!" I found myself saying cheerily, not as brave as Marie is.

"Anyway, what that means is," continued Marie, "I'll be needing quite a strong breakfast tea, and my friend here would like a peppermint tea and could you bring us some toast in case we feel like eating something?"

"Yes, of course," said the waitress. "Is there anything else I can get for you?"

"Just some water, please," I added.

"No problem."

The waitress was absolutely lovely to us, and we did eat the toast, and no one threw up or collapsed on the table. Coping with illness is often so much less dramatic than we fear it might be. Especially if we are prone to thinking about the worst case scenario.

Being with Marie and having a cup of tea and a gentle chat didn't make my migraine feel better but it made *me* feel better. Friends who understand even a little bit about your migraines will bolster you and keep you connected with the world outside pain. And friends who really understand will empathise with you and even advocate for you, making you feel less alone. It's so important because pain and illness can be incredibly isolating.

For me, Marie often acts as a role model of how not to be ashamed of my illness. She is my poster girl for flagging it up, letting people know and asking for help if needed. We don't always need the attention this brings and we can't always make the stretch to be the spokesperson. But every time we mention these types of struggles to the outside world, we maybe make it a little better not only for ourselves but for someone else. I take my dark glasses off to Marie for that.

Migraine diary and pain scale

Do yourself a favour and keep a diary of your migraines. Even though my own migraine diary, kept faithfully since 2018, records some 750 migraine episodes, I can still be surprised at how horrible a migraine feels. This is because our clever brains try their best not to store unpleasant memories about how much things hurt. You will forget how many migraines you had, when exactly you had them, what you took if anything and when they finally went away. And also, to a degree, how they felt.

I use an app called Headache Log[xxi] which, despite its name, is really well set up for migraine data. But there are loads out there and you should be able to find one you like the look of and can use easily. If you're a paper and pen person, that's just as good. Figure out what you want to record and how, and keep your diary with you as much as possible.

The diary will help you to spot patterns, if there are any. I think if I had done this in my younger years, when I got fewer migraines, I would have proved what I intuitively knew: that the migraines I did get were connected to my period in some way. Maybe I would have figured out if I was more vulnerable to a PMS migraine or an end-of-period migraine, and have some idea how long they typically lasted (so that I could count down the hours to likely freedom).

What I've discovered with my perimenopausal migraines is that there are no patterns. Literally none. It's a huge muddle of random chaos. There's no pattern with the timing of onset, the duration or the spaces between migraines. My app tells me that my average attack lasts 9 hours, but my shortest recorded migraine is 1.5 hours (an occasion where medication worked as fast as I could possibly hope) and my longest is 17 days. I've had every duration in between. Sometimes I get a two week break to recover, sometimes just a day or two before the next one hits.

In more random fun, my left and right side are similarly affected, with 340 migraines on my left side and 370 on my right. The remainder switched sides during the attack. I've taken paracetamol and ibuprofen roughly the same number of times (just shy of 300 each) and the OTC codeine tablets about the same number of times. Shockingly, I've taken triptans only 60 times. Despite it being the best drug available to me, it's the one I'm most reticent about taking. I think that's the "I must save this for the 6 days in the month I *really* need it" mentality. It often means I don't take it at all. However, I find it psychologically helpful to know I have a small stash. I think that might even be more calming for me than taking them all and actually getting the intended benefit.

In my notes, I can see that I use the phrase "no luck" as much as "took it down a notch" and "worked like a charm". The same drug regime is equally likely to result in no impact, partial impact or completely successful impact. I can have total success with a plain old ibuprofen one day, and no success at all the next. It took me ages to learn that the same was true the other way around: just because the simple solution did nothing yesterday, doesn't mean it won't work like magic today. It really feels like luck.

I felt sure if I could just work out the right combination of drugs at the correct times (a paracetamol taken at the first sign of pain; an ibuprofen taken as soon as it starts to come back) then I would "crack" this and have a fail-safe formula for dealing with any attack. But it doesn't work this way for me – not even with triptans. A triptan always makes me feel much much worse for at least fifteen minutes (as sick as I ever feel plus a ramp up of the pain) and sometimes as much as two hours. After that random amount of time, I will generally feel a slow reduction in pain and nausea, which may reach a point of no pain at all, but frequently leaves me with some pain that is manageable. This makes it worth taking, but not the fail-safe answer I was hoping for.

Keeping a migraine diary made it more transparent that there was a lot of randomness and there really wasn't a fail-safe solution. I think if I hadn't written it all down in the app, I might still be accusing myself of not trying hard enough to crack the migraine code.

I think there is probably a hit and miss element to most migraines, but perhaps perimenopausal migraines are doubly tricky. We don't understand migraines well; we don't understand perimenopause well either. Perhaps we will in the future but, for now, there is a lot of guesswork. The hormones of perimenopause, as we know, behave unpredictably. The migraines they cause therefore are also quite fickle.

It's not ideal, but it helps to know that's the case.

I also found using the pain scale in my migraine diary helped me formulate a plan for caring for myself. Firstly, it reminded me to check in with myself in a very specific way. Instead of suffering vaguely under the heading of "ugh it's a migraine" I was able to place a value on it. "This one's probably a 7 out of 10 right now, pretty tricky but not as bad as yesterday when it was a 9. I'll medicate and see if it changes. If it stays at a 9 I'll have to go and lie down." All pain values are going to be subjective, and I'm sure we all feel pain more acutely on days when we're tired, stressed or something else is going on, but nonetheless it felt empowering to slap a number on it.

Here is how I think of the pain scale specifically with regard to migraine and what my actions tend to be at each increment:

0 (No pain): I'm migraine free! Obviously I skip everywhere strewing flowers and kissing kittens.

1 (Very mild pain): Perhaps there's a very slight suggestion that I might develop a migraine sometime in the next few hours. No problem to watch and wait.

2 (Mild pain): Maybe the pain is asserting itself a bit, but it's still very manageable and I will just wait and see.

3 (Mild pain): The pain is a little irritating. This is the point at which I try to grab the simple painkillers, in the belief that medicating early can sometimes divert a migraine attack completely.

4 (Fairly moderate pain): Annoying pain. It's present but I can continue all daily activities, even though they might require more of a stretch. Another good point at which to grab those simple painkillers.

5 (Moderate pain): It's beginning to ruin my day at this point. I am really aware of the pain and have to make an effort to distract myself. Some tasks, like screenwork, are gruelling. Noise and light begin to get bothersome. If I haven't taken simple painkillers yet, I definitely will at this point.

6 (Moderate with bells and whistles): I'm really in migraine territory here. Whichever side the pain is on will be throbbing or pulsing and I'm likely to begin feeling sick. Quiet tasks are helpful and keep me distracted; noisy and/or complicated stuff will make things worse. I will consider taking an OTC medication with codeine in it.

7 (Serious pain): My head is pounding, but it is still possible to do quiet things as long as I don't go too fast. This is my cut off point for driving: I am not fit not drive at a 7. I will take an OTC codeine medication at this point.

8 (Severe pain): The pain is bad enough that my cognitive processes are affected. The pain feels hot, piercing and is impossible to ignore. I shouldn't work at this level, though I have done lots of times. Really I'm only fit to do very gentle and very quiet things. Sleep will be disrupted and it will be difficult to eat.

9 (Really severe pain): The pain is intense and it is impossible to get meaningful relief. Pain dominates my thoughts and movement is impaired/challenging. I cannot work or do more than a very simple task. I can't eat or sleep very much. I feel overwhelmed, anxious and desperate.

10 (Excruciating pain): No chance of doing anything except lying still with eyes shut. Getting to the toilet or taking a sip of water is a huge mission. No possibility of sleeping or eating at all. Even breathing feels quite tricky – the pain takes my breath away. Cognitive distortions are at their worst: I often feel convinced that I am going to have permanent brain damage, lose one of my eyes or even die. Light and noise are unbearable.

    A migraine attack can begin anywhere on the pain scale. Some folk begin with no pain at all, but disturbances in their vision or a feeling or sudden fatigue give them the clue that a migraine isn't far off. For me, pain is my first symptom. That can mean a mild pain that I'd rate somewhere between 1 and 3, or it can start as a 4 or 5. Sometimes, it will rush in at a higher score, but usually only if I've done something to aggravate it like accidentally look into a car headlight at night or broken into a sprint for some reason. Commonly, I will get milder pain first and it will gradually ramp up over an hour or two until it's a full-on migraine. Knowing this helps me to plan to take those simple painkillers early on in the process, which can stop the worst of the pain from arriving at all.

Thankfully, I've only hit a 10 on the pain scale 15 times since I started keeping my migraine diary. It's helped to realise, through my records, that the very worst pain is rare (2% of the time). I've hit a 9 some 43 times, which happens three times as often as a 10, and accounts for 6% of my migraines. I've recorded a pain score of 8 for 75 attacks, which is 10% of them. I know I shouldn't be at work while it's this bad, but I understand why I have pushed myself through it. If I stop working at level 8, I cancel a lot more sessions than if my cut-off is 9 and above. I don't have the data for how many sessions I would have cancelled if that had been my policy, but it's probably safe to say my business would have suffered.

My diary shows that my migraine pain is severe or worse just under a fifth of the time. That means that four-fifths of the time, my pain might be limiting but it is manageable. Levels 4-7 aren't fun, but they don't seem to affect my thinking, and that in itself means I have more resources at my disposal to work with the pain. At 4-7, I can reason very competently about pain and its management. At level 8 and above my judgement is clouded by fear as my body goes into emergency mode. At the most basic level, when pain is severe, we think something must be very wrong. We are hardwired to get that message. It helps to be aware that that's what's going on, but it doesn't mean it's possible to override the message. I'm glad I'm only in that state for a fifth of my attacks.

My diary cleverly works out and displays my average pain score on its homepage, and it's been interesting to see it change. It used to be a 7, pretty solidly. Sometime in the past year or so, it's dropped to a 6. That's still moderate pain with bells and whistles, of course, but it helps to see that my scores are going down.

There's also a great calendar view which enables me to see at a glance that my attacks are getting fewer, with longer gaps between them. Now and then there's a blip and I'll have a monster attack that lasts 5 days and feels awful, but it's helpful to be able to set that into a larger and more optimistic picture.

My friend, Marie, had an interesting response when I shared with her that things seemed to be going in a hopeful direction. She said "Be prepared for the chance that the migraines might never go away." She wasn't being a party pooper. She was simply saying, I think, beware taking too much hope from the data trends. Just because the numbers go in the direction we want, doesn't mean they will keep doing so. Perimenopausal hormones are punk rockers, remember. And hormones are a bit punk rock, period. The numbers may not keep going in a beautiful trajectory down to zero. There may be level 6s for life, and I may never be safe from a 10 on the pain scale for some percentage of the time.

But here, the diary comes to my rescue again. It says, implicitly, in every entry, that I have got through it. 750 odd times. And I will again.

Sleep

As you'll know if you have migraines, you cannot "sleep it off". I have told myself I will "probably sleep it off" so many times and the truth is the only time you actually sleep it off is when you're right at the tail end of a migraine, going into the hangover/recovery phase. Then you will be pretty exhausted and sleep will finally be possible and so, so welcome.

But during any other part of a migraine attack, don't kid yourself.

There is great value in pairing the taking of your medication of choice with a lie down. I highly recommend it. It doesn't matter whether you've got a bit of a nagging pain so you've decided to get in early with an ibuprofen, or you're at your wits end with a banger and you're waiting for a triptan to kick in. If you go and lie down in a dark room in complete silence, you'll give yourself a better shot.

However, it's just not always possible, is it? It's so frequently impossible, because *life*, that I just have to accept that I'm going to lower my odds of the migraine shifting more readily by doing something other than going for a lie down. And have you tried lying down during the day? See how long you can do it before you get interrupted by a delivery, a phonecall, a power tool, a bin lorry, a cat fight, etc. Don't even get me started on streaks of sunlight having the audacity to come through the curtains.

If you do commit to a lie down, go all out. Silence your phone. Use a bulldog clip or two to ensure your curtains stay shut, or don an eye mask. Put ear plugs in or noise cancelling headphones on. Tell whoever you live with that you need half an hour of silence, uninterrupted. If you live with small people, lower your expectations. If you live with older children and adults, they should be able to turn their TV/games console down and resist slamming doors for 30 minutes. If they still won't hush their beaks, and they are related to you by blood, remind them that migraine is very heritable, and you would hate to join a brass band just as they experience their first migraine attacks, but you bloody well will if they force your hand.

During the worst migraine attacks, you won't be able to sleep, but you can try to rest. It is terribly difficult to remain in a calm enough state to rest when you are in the upper echelons of the pain scale, but you can attempt it with some deep breaths and gentle reminders that you really are safe. On a physical level, it helps if your bed is comfortable and your clothes are loose and layered. On a mental level, some gentle mind games can help take away the worst of the panic stricken thought galloping.

I have three such mind games tucked away that work for me. If they work for you, nab them. If not, there are loads more ideas along these lines. Experiment.

The first is the alphabet game. You'll know it. Pick a category (an easy one: you've got a migraine) and think of a word beginning with each letter of the alphabet in that category. It's just taxing enough to keep your anxious mind from flying off in a thousand other directions, without actually being that taxing. Oh, and don't expect yourself to actually be able to *do* the game. Your migraine brain will have you losing whole sections of the alphabet, reassigning letters all over the show and not being able to remember what things start with. The point is not to play the game well but to distract your poor anxious mind and maybe even bore yourself to sleep.

The second is that I imagine a house or an apartment, quite a lovely one probably, but empty and painted white. I go through it in my mind and decorate it any way I see fit, arranging the furniture and fittings of my choice however I like, and accessorising to my heart's content. All the fun of home renovation without any of the stress. Again, a little engaging, but not too much. Rooms can be left in any state of unfinishedness you want. Every single room I've ever imaginary decorated while migraining has been a dark, lying down room that smells of peppermint and has a water supply at arm's reach.

And the third one is to time travel back to nice places I've been. A quiet beach with warm waves and shade from nearby trees. The vast lobby of a place we once stayed that had really cosy sofas and dim lighting and a huge open fire. A forest I've taken autumnal walks through. Make it whatever is pleasant for you, whatever gives you small pieces of joy. The point is not wild excitement (which doesn't mix well with migraines) but comfort and ease (which does).

It's hard to fill nighttimes of fitful wakefulness while you are kept awake by migraine. The hours really stretch, and we are all more vulnerable to anxiety in the small hours, in the dark, never mind when you throw head pain into the mix as well. Treat yourself as kindly as you can.

The other thing to say about sleep is that it can be preventative. That is, if you can get into a good sleep routine when you are well, you may suffer fewer migraines. Lack of sleep is a trigger for me, for sure, as is not sleeping at my usual times. If I'm even off by half an hour, sometimes that will be enough to cause a migraine.

Sleep, when it is regular and restful, has a myriad of benefits for both physical and mental health. Matthew Walker has written an excellent book called *Why We Sleep* all about it – if you need any more convincing, get yourself a copy. But, in short, most adults need between 7 and 9 hours of sleep per night. I feel best with a solid 8 most of the time, though after a bad migraine I need 9 for at least a couple of nights.

When I am well, I am tired by 9:30pm (yeah, I'm middle aged, it's fine), in bed reading by 10pm and usually sound asleep between 10:30 and 11pm. Then I'll generally feel alright about getting up between 6:30 and 7am. So I've got really boring about it. I don't vary my routine much. It means I get all the sleep I need when I am migraine-free, even if I don't get that luxury during an attack. It may prevent some of my migraines, but some of them are coming for me anyway, no matter how diligent I am.

I think it may mean I have more resilience in the bank when a migraine hits. Everyone knows that the better rested you are, the better you can cope. That's certainly true of coping with migraine attacks. If I've had a few nights of decent sleep before one hits, there's a little more in the tank. Also, sleeping well at the tail end of a migraine is very healing. It can take a few nights to feel that I've fully recovered, but ensuring those nights adhere to my usual sleep routine (or even getting into my pit a little early) really helps.

Caffeine

It's well known that caffeine can trigger migraines. This is because your body quickly adjusts to the level of caffeine you put in it, and would ideally like you to put the same amount in at the same times each day (or give it a little more – but, crucially, not too much less). If it misses its regular fix, it will kick off, and one of the things you might experience is a caffeine withdrawal headache or migraine.

The caffeine withdrawal migraine is a nasty thing, giving you plenty enough pain and nausea to have you reaching for the nearest caffeinated beverage post haste. This makes caffeine very hard to give up.

Also, different people are differently sensitive to variations in their daily caffeine intake. Some might vary their intake by quite a lot and not notice much difference, because their bodies happen not to be very sensitive to caffeine. Others might find that someone accidentally making their regular 11am latte decaf sends them into a pit of migraine hell by noon. This may go hand in hand with their overall sensitivity to caffeine: we all know people who can sup espresso just before falling asleep. Other people find it impacts their sleep so negativity they don't drink it after a certain time of day, or at all.

One of the things caffeine does, alongside improving our alertness, is to narrow our blood vessels and reduce blood flow (a neat little trick called vasoconstriction)[xxii]. One of the causes of headaches and migraines is dilated blood vessels in the brain – it's thought the increased blood flow can contribute to migraine's characteristic thumping or pounding sensation[xxiii]. In fact, this is one of the things triptans do: they reverse this dilation in the brain's blood vessels using vasoconstriction. Caffeine does this in a less dramatic way, which is why some OTC branded painkillers also contain caffeine – it speeds up your absorption of the painkiller and helpfully does a bit of vasoconstriction to ease that throbbing. (You can recreate the effect more cheaply by taking your generic paracetamol or ibuprofen with your caffeinated drink of choice).

While it isn't a good idea to over-caffeinate yourself (whole host of horrible health problems can result), and while you should definitely bear in mind what you think your own personal limit is according to your own sensitivity to it, I have found that a little bit of caffeine is a helpful thing for migraines.

I love nice coffee and tea, and in the past I have definitely perked myself up a little during migraine attacks by having one or the other. Especially when taken with painkillers, it did seem to aid my ability to cope and sometimes to speed up recovery time. This was probably a combination of the mild stimulant effect alongside the vasoconstriction.

It also didn't go amiss during the migraine recovery period.

However, a couple of years ago, due to developing an arrhythmia, I had to give up caffeine. It was a blow to give up tea and coffee but I tried to look on the bright side: if it really did trigger migraines in any way, perhaps I would now experience fewer of them?

I can confirm that the lack of caffeine made no difference whatsoever. Still as many migraines, still as bad, still ever so random. And now, no chance of boosting my vasoconstriction with a nice cup of tea.

So, if you look at your migraine diary and you see no unhelpful correlation between your migraines and caffeine, don't feel you have to give it up. It may actually be aiding your recovery.

But if you do find caffeine is a trigger, or you just want to give it up for other reasons, here are my tips for you:

- Reduce your caffeine consumption slowly rather than going cold turkey: this will prevent the awful caffeine withdrawal migraine from being so bad.
- Experiment with decaf coffees and teas and find a few you like. I really missed nice coffee and tea and finding some decent decaf alternatives helped a lot with that.
- However, lower your expectations. Decaf coffee and tea, even though I promise you will adjust to it and even think it's quite nice, is never going to be as good as the caffeinated version.
- Remember that lots of soft drinks contain caffeine, not just the obvious ones. Read your labels.
- Do yourself a favour on so many levels (not just those relating to caffeine) and don't touch energy drinks or weight loss supplements. They almost always contain a shedload of caffeine.

And one last thing on caffeine: you can also find it in chocolate. So yes, you can eat chocolate to help your migraine (sadly you may not feel like eating chocolate while you have a migraine, which is classic Sod's Law isn't it?) There's more in dark chocolate than milk chocolate, and none in white chocolate, so bear that in mind when selecting your chocolatey medicine. There is also only about 30% of the caffeine in a small bar of milk chocolate that there is in your average cup of builder's tea, so it's a really small amount. This is the reason that neither my migraines nor my arrhythmia have parted me from my favourite chocolate.

Water

You don't need me to tell you that you must drink water, especially when you have a migraine.

But the reality is that it won't be easy to drink even water when your head is pounding and you feel like you're going to throw up. Remember, your whole body will go into emergency mode and forget about luxury processes like absorption and digestion, so any water you do manage to drink will sit high up in your stomach and make you feel even more likely to vomit at any moment. You will generally feel better – or at least be convinced you do – with an empty stomach, while your migraine is really bad.

Therefore, get the water in early. At the first gnawing of pain, start drinking more water than you usually do. Other fluids count too, but you really can't beat water for hydration with no added extras to complicate things. If your pee starts looking nice and pale, you're doing a great job, and you should keep it up for as long as you can.

If the attack gets really bad though, and you can't face the thought of swallowing anything, try to make water the exception. You can go without food for a little while without too much ill effect, but going without water is going to slow down your recovery – and, eventually, put a lot of other stresses on your body.

One trick I've used if I'm in so much pain that I'm just lying in a dark room trying to remember to breathe, is to drink a sip of water every five minutes. By the time it's this bad, you have little else to do except wonder how you can be in this much pain and not actually die, so it can help make the hours crawl by just slightly less torturously.

Another trick is to drink peppermint tea. Peppermint helps a little with nausea (it's no magic bullet, but it can take the edge off temporarily) and it can be comforting to have a hot drink. I can get quite cold when I have a migraine so the prospect of a hot drink encourages me to drink a little faster and a little more. It's also not horrible cold, so if you can't manage to drink it at a rate swifter than one sip per five minutes, it's not wasted.

Drink more water than usual when you're out the other side and recovering from the migraine, too: it will help you to combat the fatigue and residual pain a little faster.

And carry water everywhere with you. Do not leave home without it in your bag. You never know when the first niggles of a migraine will begin, or when you'll need to take a painkiller. It will get you in the habit of hydrating no matter where you are and what you're doing, which is a good thing for all sorts of reasons.

The downside of all this healthy water consumption is that you will need to pee a lot. I have developed an encyclopaedic knowledge of the whereabouts of every public toilet in my home town. I go through life marvelling at people who can suggest an impromptu picnic in the park, because these are clearly people who skip through life with empty bladders and yet no migraine pain to consider.

Food

You won't want to eat when you have a migraine that hits 8 and above on the pain scale. It's just out of the question. Try not to worry about this, as long as you are drinking water. Try to drink other things if you can – things with a bit of sugar in, to give you just the barest boost of energy. Maybe you can stand a cup of herbal tea with a spoonful of honey stirred into it – that will do.

And once the pain comes down, nourish yourself with care. Start simple with some toast, some eggs, maybe a bowl of cereal or a jacket potato. Then, as soon as that settles and you feel like it, ensure you get all your regular meals and snacks and, of course, plenty of water. You are likely to feel weak, shaky and exhausted. Sometimes frequent, smaller meals and snacks for a day or two can really help with that. Try to get some calorie dense foods to make up for all the nutrition you missed while you were too ill to eat: peanut butter sandwiches are a good bet, maybe some pasta in a cheese sauce, a smoothie with some full fat yoghurt and an avocado (plus, you know, some other stuff to make it taste nice) or nuts and dried fruit for snacking. For a lot of people, a bit of caffeine is helpful: there's nothing more comforting than a cup of tea and a few squares of chocolate, is there?

You may find that there's a food you can eat while you're really ill, either because it doesn't make you want to throw up, or it's actually not the worst thing in the world to throw up if it comes to that. For me, that food is bananas. I can nearly always manage to nibble a banana, actually even when my pain's been at a 9. But, as you know, I can usually trust my nausea not to turn to vomiting, which does help. Ginger biscuits are another food that I can generally manage at least a little of, and toast is my go-to recovery food. Little pieces of crystallised ginger, which you can source in health food shops, can also temporarily relieve nausea sometimes.

Migraines tend to cause constipation, because the body slows down during an attack, and digestion can be really sluggish. Add in that we're struggling to drink as much as we should, or move as much as we normally do, and it's hardly surprising that migraine sufferers might not poo regularly during attacks. If you medicate with codeine, it's well known that codeine causes constipation too, though I have found that migraines constipate me whether I use codeine or not.

Things return to their normal rhythm once the worst of the migraine has passed, and you can help things along by ensuring you drink water and include enough fruit, vegetables and other fibre in your recovery meals.

I tend to find myself craving foods I know and foods that are relatively plain, which makes sense. My poor system is thrown all over the place as I sometimes eat nothing, sometimes eat well, sometimes get constipated, sometimes feel like my stomach is delicate...no wonder it wants no extra surprises.

During those times when there is either no migraine or the pain level is lower, I find that eating regularly is very helpful. The food itself doesn't seem to matter that much – I don't find that there's any particular food that either triggers or helps a migraine – but not getting too hungry does make a difference. By the time I'm starving hungry and ready to eat the first thing I see, I've usually got the beginnings of a migraine as well.

Eating regularly enough that I don't get too hungry means, for me, eating three meals a day plus three snacks. I get hungry all the bloody time. I think I'm just one of those people who feels better eating little and often (or, truthfully, lots and still fairly often). Along with drinking my water, this feels like one of the best tools in my armoury for preventing a migraine.

It's also surprised me how much food helps when I am on the pain scale anywhere up to an 8. It seems counter-intuitive, but I often find my pain score goes down by as much as 2 or 3 while I am eating and for a short while afterwards. It seems to really help with nausea as well. I might feel quite sick but, after one bite of toast, the feeling has vanished. It will return with a vengeance in about half an hour, mind you, but the respite is really nice.

If you are someone who experiences nausea and vomiting with your migraines, and nothing you do with your diet during an attack seems to help, do not suffer in silence. If you are going days without being able to eat (some poor folk can't even keep water down) your body will be really struggling and recovering from an attack becomes that much harder. See your GP about anti-nausea medication (anti-emetics) that you can take alongside a painkiller or a triptan (and will hopefully stop you throwing up your precious pain meds, too). If you can't swallow *anything*, not even an anti-nausea pill – oh, the irony – then some of these meds can be given as suppositories. I can't imagine shoving stuff up your butt feels brilliant when you're on the verge of puking, either, but needs must.

I am not a believer in following some prescribed diet for migraine, though fair play to you if you find subsisting on organic tofu and kale helps. The one time I did an elimination diet (for reasons other than migraine) and had to live on just meat, fish and veggies for two weeks, I felt absolutely abysmal: weak, shaky and generally awful. The moment I was allowed to include bread again I felt so much better, not to mention getting back dairy and chocolate.

One thing is for sure if you have migraines: intermittent fasting is not for you. Might as well call it intermittent migraines. In my experience, intermittent fasting increases the frequency and the severity of the migraines, and is not worth messing with.

I know I have to eat my vegetables and salad, but they are not the things that make me feel my best – I feel good instantly after eating a marmite sandwich and a KitKat. So I try to balance the things that make me feel good with the things that I know are good for me. I know a lot of people struggle with this (me included) and I've found the best way to think about it is to decide what you'd feed a child you want the best for, and then feed yourself (adult portions of) that.

Alcohol

Alcohol is a trigger for many people with migraines, partly because it's so good at dehydrating us and partly because it contains a bunch of chemicals that may be implicated in migraine pain[xxiv]. Some people find they can't drink red wine, or beer, but other types of alcohol are fine, and others find that they can't really drink more than a very small amount of alcohol before a migraine arrives.

I think because my migraines are linked to hormones, alcohol was an unpredictable trigger for me. Sometimes I could drink in quite large quantities and be unbothered, and other times one glass of wine would bring a migraine on. Frequently, a hangover headache would morph into a migraine – maybe one I would have had anyway, or maybe not.

The problem was, I really loved my alcohol. It was a major part of my social life and I told myself it was also how I liked to wind down. It was a treat after a tough day, a celebration after a great day, a pick me up if I was lacking energy and a relaxation aid if I was stressed. I had attributed many magical properties to alcohol, some of which were quite conflicting, and I was ignoring the inconvenient truth that sometimes it triggered migraines and sometimes the hangovers were awful.

I am not proud of this, but I used to use my migraine medication as a free pass to keep drinking. Especially in the early days of my perimenopausal migraines, when the painkillers reliably took the pain away, I medicated instead of stopping drinking. Or I drank freely, knowing that if the next day's hangover grew hairy and large, I could pop a couple of strong painkillers to take the edge off it. I told myself that this was me being determined not to miss out on life, and that this was therefore a totally legitimate use of my medication. The fact was, I saw alcohol as an integral part of my life that I really didn't want to let go of.

I thought I was the life and soul of the party on alcohol, but the truth was that sometimes I couldn't remember what I had done or how I had behaved. I also thought no one could really tell when I was drunk (at the same time as believing it turned me into the life and soul of the party) until my daughter got a bit older and definitely began to spot when I'd had three glasses of wine with dinner. My husband, always a moderate drinker who could take it or leave it, would also know full well I was squiffy. He never made a fuss about it, but more than once he picked up the pieces when I lost my shit over something or other and ended up crying on him. I'm actually good at dealing with emotions – I've made a career out of it – but not, most definitely not, when I've been drinking.

I knew I didn't like my drunkenness, and increasingly I didn't like myself hungover. Not only did my head pound the whole of the next day, along with the expected nausea and tiredness, but I also began to feel incredibly anxious. Some of this was directly related to the drinking: I worried over what I'd done, who I'd upset and what people had noticed. But some of it seemed to come out of nowhere. It was general anxiety and it's common to experience an upsurge during perimenopause, but this seemed to always hit me harder on a hangover day (or, increasingly, for a couple of days after drinking heavily).

Still, it wasn't as easy as realising it was doing me no good and giving it up: I still held fast to the narrative that alcohol helped me to be more social, be more relaxed, be more lively, be more me. It didn't make sense to give up something I still thought of as a treat.

In the end, there was no big moment that made me give it up. No big disastrous night out (though there had been many smaller disasters along the way) and no particularly horrendous hangover. Just a slight cold during the 2021 lockdown that made me crave hot tea and warm blankets several nights in a row, and a daughter upset by missing her friends while school was closed who needed my full presence, and then amazingly I hadn't had a drink for a whole week, and I wondered if I could go another week, and it turned out I could.

It didn't seem to make a difference to the migraines. They still came thick and fast and were as bad as ever. But it made a massive difference to my anxiety. That certainly reduced, but also when it was there, I could deal with it. Of course I could deal with it: I help other people deal with anxiety every day, I could definitely put my mind to helping myself just as effectively (more on exactly how, below). I just needed a clear head to do it, that was all.

And I hadn't appreciated how much anxiety alcohol itself caused me. While there was an open bottle of wine in the fridge, my mind kept returning to when I would drink it, how much of it I would drink, how I could get away with draining the rest of the bottle. Or I would be thinking about the next "good excuse" to make a gin and tonic, or whether or not I fancied a beer, or whether it was high time for a nightcap. When sharing booze with others, I wouldn't be able to relax until it was all poured, waiting for my next top up, assessing how buzzed I was and finding I was never quite buzzed enough.

I could not understand friends who nursed one drink all evening, or – mystifying! – could leave some alcohol in their glass. I get it now: they were enjoying their drink, and they knew when they'd had enough, or else they were so neutral about drinking it didn't matter to them if they didn't finish every last drop. After I gave up drinking I saw that drinking was not like that for me, and I didn't think it ever would be. I never ever drank a glass of anything to enjoy it for its own sake. I drank to get drunk. Even if I stopped at one, I was thinking about what it would be like to have six and get wasted. Most of the time, I didn't get completely wasted, but I was managing that constant tension of thinking maybe I wanted to be. It was a relief to give that up.

Not drinking at all is just easier for me. I no longer have to negotiate that boundary with alcohol. I thought I would miss it or crave it or be tempted to "just have one", but it hasn't been like that. I've simply felt a weight come off me for giving myself permission not to engage with it at all.

It turns out that I don't need it to be sociable, and at least I remember the social interactions I had now and feel more in control of them. It also turns out that I relax much better without wine in my system, and that I'm far more capable of managing any emotion sober than I was tipsy. I sleep better and I feel less anxious. It may not have made a big dent in the migraines, but there have been so many big wins for me from cutting alcohol out that I doubt I'll ever go back to it, even if there comes a day when migraines are a thing of the past.

Managing stress

Stress is not the only cause of migraines, but it can make them worse. In terms of perimenopausal migraines, stress influences what hormones do, so there is a connection. Having said that, I've had stressful times where I haven't had a migraine, as well as stressful times that have brought on a thumper. I've also had plenty of migraines when I wasn't stressed. However, I think it'd be remiss not to look into the connection and try to work with it.

My poor Dad used to get migraines on weekends sometimes after a stressful week at work. It was awful timing – he'd just had five days of pressure with deadlines, and would be looking forward to a bit of respite, when a migraine would arrive and see him having to stay in bed for the whole of Saturday and Sunday. This is a common pattern for stress-induced migraines: they leave you alone while you're going through the actual stress, and then knock you for six the minute you start to calm down and relax. This is known as a "let-down" headache or migraine, and it due to cortisol levels fluctuating[xxv]. Cortisol is a hormone that lends a hand when we need it, usually in times of stress. It can reduce any pain or inflammation and generally aid us in getting on with stuff when things get demanding. However, it's only supposed to be for short term use. If it fluctuates over the course of a day, for example, getting a boost when you need to run for the bus and then levelling out for much of the rest of the time, that's not a problem. If your stressful demands continue over a longer period, and your cortisol levels remain elevated, it's harder on your body when you do experience fluctuation. You fall harder, and further. That explains why some people get migraines at the start of a weekend or holiday, or just after a period of stress.

Cortisol also impacts other hormones. When women of menstruating age are going through something particularly stressful, it's not uncommon for them to skip ovulation or even miss a period. This is because cortisol affects our oestrogen and progesterone levels[xxvi]. Usually, when the stress goes away, the menstrual cycle returns to normal too.

So what about during perimenopause, when our hormones are going haywire anyway? Well, this is the time when our ovaries, previously the powerhouses of oestrogen production, wind down their work. Oestrogen is produced in diminishing quantities, and mainly by the adrenal glands instead of the ovaries. Adrenal glands are also where our stress hormones, like cortisol and adrenaline, are being produced. So if the adrenal glands are really busy pumping out loads of stress hormones, they put stuff like oestrogen on the backburner.

And we already know, from our general merrily hellish experience of perimenopause, that adjusting to less oestrogen is a toughie. It's responsible for so many troublesome perimenopausal symptoms, including migraines. So, the more stressed we are, the less our bodies are able to focus on chucking some oestrogen our way every now and then to help us out.

But the pickle remains: how do we deal with stress? In midlife it's not unusual for women to be doing well in their careers while raising a family and possibly caring for ageing parents or relatives, which is quite enough of a load to cause stress. Add into that what we know about trauma causing stress reactions well after the event, and it's a wonder any of us has a low cortisol level.

I mention trauma because it disproportionately affects women. One in 4 women experiences domestic violence, 1 in 9 experiences childhood sexual abuse and 1 in 4 are raped[xxvii] (these are UK statistics, but they give you some clue as to the numbers of women who are dealing with trauma related to assault or sexual assault). A meta analysis of a number of studies showed that people with childhood trauma are more at risk for developing migraine, as are people with PTSD or CPTSD[xxviii].

This is because stressful experiences can change the way our limbic system works. The limbic system is an area of the brain that controls emotions, behaviour and memory so, if it changes due to traumatic events, it can work less effectively[xxix].

If your cortisol levels were skyrocketing because you were coping with abuse as a youngster, it can be hard to even know what a baseline level of stress hormones feels like. If you were constantly on high alert because your childhood was a dangerous place, you may have to learn as an adult what safety actually feels like.

Of course, if you experience something traumatic like sexual violence as an adult, your previously steady view of the world (and your stress response to it) can also change radically, and permanently[xxx]. It's not uncommon for people to become hypervigilant, that is, on the lookout for terrible things to happen again. Such constant hypervigilance, especially against something that we ultimately don't get to control, raises cortisol levels but also can leave us in a sensitive state where things like pain affect us more[xxxi]. In other words, we are not just training ourselves to be vigilant to danger, but vigilant to everything – and pain can be a signal that danger is on the way, so it makes sense we'd feel it more.

It can feel hopeless to believe that we are suffering double: we already went through the trauma, and now we're getting migraines too. But managing the responses to trauma can be done. It won't cure your perimenopausal migraine: your hormones are still going to cause trouble. But they might just cause a bit less trouble, on a less regular basis.

Trauma therapy is a specific type of therapy that comprises several different strands of treatment. This should always be practised by a therapist specially trained in trauma. I trained for four years to be a therapist but I am not a trauma specialist and I am not qualified to lead this kind of complex work. However, through my work I know of excellent practitioners who do this, often with great results.

You don't have to find a specialist, and incur the expense of that, necessarily. You can get yourself on an NHS waiting list, but you won't be offered specialist trauma therapy unless you are severely affected – the thresholds for accessing this are very high. However, ordinary talk therapy can get you a long way, if you can find a therapist you simply feel comfortable with.

This is what I did. I experienced childhood trauma, CSA and also an isolated incidence of sexual violence in my teens. I was by no means the most severe case out there, but talk therapy in my twenties helped me enormously and I only wished I'd done it sooner. I felt I could tell my therapist anything and she listened attentively, always making me feel understood. The magic of that helped me deal with a great deal of emotional pain and to develop good ways to continue processing it. It was a large part of the reason that I became a therapist myself, and I still don't hesitate to return to therapy whenever I need it.

Therapy is an unregulated industry in the UK. This means that anyone can call themselves a counsellor or therapist and take your money – they don't have to had any training at all, and this is perfectly legal (though definitely morally questionable). To protect yourself, always search for a therapist who belongs to a reputable organisation for professional therapists – in the UK, the main ones are the British Association of Counsellors and Psychotherapists (BACP) and the UK Council for Psychotherapy (UKCP). You can be sure that anyone listed on their directories is fully qualified to practise.

Of course, that doesn't necessarily mean they'll be a good therapist or the right therapist for you. There's a certain amount of just having to meet them and see if it feels right. Don't feel obliged to stay for more sessions if a first, second or third session doesn't feel right. There are lots of therapists out there: keep going until you find one you feel completely comfortable with.

If money is an issue there are usually organisations in larger towns and cities that offer a sliding scale or lower rates. Have a look around and ask for recommendations. In addition, a great many therapists in private practice offer some sessions at lower rates. It's worth contacting them to see if they have anything at a rate you can manage.

NHS therapy usually means a long wait and then a set number of sessions, and no choice of therapist or therapeutic approach. The NHS tends to employ CBT practitioners because there is a lot of evidence for the efficacy of CBT – it's the mode of therapy that's easiest to measure. CBT is structured and therapist-led, which suits a great many people, especially if they want something specific e.g. strategies to work with anxious thoughts, or improving sleep. It's not the best modality for working with multiple or more complex issues. This is where I think a humanistic approach, which is client centred, can be more helpful. This style of therapy is unstructured and puts the emphasis on the client talking about whatever is painful while the therapist closely tracks them and communicates their empathy and understanding. Through this process, the client usually figures out some possible ways forward, which the therapist helps them to explore and put into practice.

I am a great advocate of humanistic therapy because it is what I practice and also what got me through all the tough stuff in my own therapy. But I do think it's horses for courses: if you want more direction, or your goals are specific, CBT will probably suit you much better.

Of course, therapy is only part of the picture when it comes to managing stress. If you go to therapy, you'll still need to manage your stress outside sessions. And if therapy isn't for you, there's a lot you can do yourself.

The place to start is a really honest inventory of what's causing you stress. You'd think this would be easy for a therapist who spends all day helping people look at stressful things, but here's a conversation I had recently with my husband about whether or not I worry about things.

"I was listening to a podcast that reminded me of you," my husband said, "because it was about people who worry about things a lot."

"But I don't worry about things too much."

Husband gives me a knowing look

"Well, OK, I do worry a lot about *some* things," I conceded.

I can get so busy managing, fixing and organising things that I forget to notice whether something is causing me stress or not. I think this is the trap of being so busy "doing" we lose what the "being" is like. It can take someone looking in from the outside to pinpoint the stress and anxiety that may be aggravating migraines.

This is where a friend or partner can be very helpful. They can sometimes see your signs of stress before you spot them, or they can question things that you brush over as "business as usual." Once you can see this potential sources of stress, you have choices around them. If you're unaware they're even causing stress, you don't.

And if you don't have someone to talk this through with (or even if you do) then writing it all down can be just as good. Write longhand if you can: it slows you down, and makes it very obviously from you. Getting the words out of your head and into the air or onto a page is the thing. Once you can see how it is, you can work with it.

Once you have your stress inventory, you have decisions to make. Some things you will be able to sling out. You perhaps didn't even realise you were still hanging onto them, they serve no benefit to you, and you'll feel better dropping them.

Some things you'll conclude are worth the stress. This is where there is some benefit to you, perhaps, or to someone you love very much, and you are prepared to take on the extra because of that. Fine. At least you're choosing it. That is an important mental shift.

But inevitably there will be some stressful things you feel you can't drop even though you'd love to, probably things you can't easily admit to out loud. This is where you find the wiggle room. Can you make these things easier on yourself so that, when you have to do them, they aren't as stressful? Sometimes this involves tweaking the logistics, sometimes this involves bringing on board extra help and sometimes this involves adjusting your own headspace. Look for the ways you can modify things to reduce your stress, even if only a bit. Part of the point of it is feeling like you have some agency.

Something else that you can look at when managing stress is to ask yourself how your internal chatter is. Do you constantly berate and criticise yourself, or do you cheer yourself on a bit? I don't need to tell you that if it's the former, you'll feel a lot more stressed. It's like trying to do difficult things while someone yells "You're bloody useless!" in your ear all day long. If you're going to do difficult things, far better to have a kinder voice accompanying you who says "Hey, you're doing your best" and "You're marvellous" and "Let's have a bath and an early night, we've earned it."

But if you're under the thumb from a critical inner voice, you'll know it's not easy to change it. It's not like changing a radio channel to something you like better. It's more like removing permanent ink from a whiteboard and painstakingly rewriting.

This is because our inner voices essentially come from childhood: they are usually a version of the people who looked after us and who we spent the most time with. If those people spent the majority of their time encouraging us and telling us we were doing alright, chances are we will absorb those messages and be able to tell ourselves that as adults, without even really thinking about it. But if those people were more critical, or didn't have time to help with our struggles, or were too preoccupied with their own struggles to see ours, then we'll have a less helpful inner chatter to contend with.

So, if your internal voice needs work, remember to be patient: you will not be able to move from critical to kind overnight. You probably won't be able to change things much at all in the beginning: you'll catch yourself often in your default critical brain chat. It helps to consciously talk kindly to yourself at least once a day in the beginning. Maybe pick a time or a part of your day that's not too stressful for you and really focus on how you're talking to yourself about it in your own head. Make an effort to talk supportively, or at least neutrally, for as long as you can (this is in your own head so no one needs to even know you're doing it, though of course you can do it out loud if you're comfortable with that and don't mind the funny looks). If you struggle, imagine what someone who loves you would say to you. If you still struggle, imagine what you'd say to someone you love, and then say that to yourself.

It might feel weird, it might feel icky, but keep doing it. This is how I started, in my twenties, when my self talk was like living with the most vitriolic, negative bitch almost 24 hours a day (yes, it even crept into my dreams). The change was so gradual that I cannot tell you exactly when I managed to be more kind than cruel to myself, but I promise you that I am very grateful to myself for just starting. To be clear, changing your chatter doesn't mean you'll have no bad and stressful days. You just won't make them even worse by scolding yourself silly about them. Even on the worst days, you'll be understanding towards yourself, even when you've done something you're not happy about. I am hardly ever a bitch to myself nowadays. And it makes life infinitely nicer.

One final thing for dealing with stress. It's kind of an anti-dealing with stress thing. I call it having moments. I don't mean senior moments, or those brain fog moments where you can't remember your own name, or even magic moments – though chocolate often comes into this for me. I mean sometimes it's a good idea to just have a little moment where you focus on nothing except what's right in front of you.

This is not the same as the advice to "live in the moment" which is just plain unworkable. Not many of us can truly dump both past and future and not have to give a thought to anything except the present. Nor do I think we really want to, honestly: the past informs how we got to the present, in varied and complex and interesting ways. And what we want from the future informs how we use the present, removing some of the anxiety that comes from the uncertainty of that future. So I certainly don't advocate for concentrating on the present moment at all costs.

But sometimes it's OK to take a break from juggling the complexities of the past, the demands of the present and the considerations of the future. There's real freedom in staring out of the window, dipping a Twix in your tea and watching the leaves fall off the trees. There's something simplifying in imagining that all you have to do for the next ten minutes is fold the laundry. That way you can notice how good it smells and how much you like your sweaters, instead of folding on autopilot whilst worrying about thirteen other things. And if you can steal away and do something that's purely, truly just for you and just because for even five minutes, it will be a real counter-stress initiative. Whether it's belting a football, picking up your knitting, playing a few rounds of MarioKart or reading a chapter of your book, just absolutely milk that moment for all it's worth.

Soon enough you will need to return to those other things, and that's OK. We all need to tend to what needs doing. But make sure you have a moment, at least once every day, that's at the least a break from thinking too much and at the best feels like a little treat.

Do things anyway

The worst thing about migraine – even worse than the crippling pain – is missing out on things. I've missed big things like birthdays and New Year celebrations, I've missed nice things like meeting up with friends and going out for dinner, I've missed work and I've missed countless small things that make up every day family life. You know, the little bits like helping with homework, baking, going on a bike ride – the bits that, added up, matter a lot.

One thing to know is that if you do the small things all the time when you're well – which you do – people will get by without you doing them when you're ill. If you have a partner, they're very capable of stepping in (and if they're not, maybe you're getting stress migraines?)

If you don't have a partner, but you have kids, let them surprise you with how capable and independent they can be, in age appropriate ways of course. My daughter is a legend at emptying dishwashers and cooking curries, which may partly be a legacy of taking over when I had a migraine. These are useful life skills and I shouldn't feel bad that she has them.

The other thing to know is that sometimes it hurts less to do things anyway. I often feel glad that I kept my plans and did the thing anyway, even if I had to modify it by not staying as long or not getting as involved.

You've got to pick and choose – the plan to attend a loud gig or meet your most stressy friend would not be first choices with a migraine. But maybe the walk round the park with your partner or visiting your friend who always makes tea and feeds you biscuits or going to the library with your kids is OK. It doesn't make you feel any worse in terms of pain, and you feel glad afterwards that you didn't have to write off your whole day.

One of my struggles with this policy is that I never know how much better or worse a migraine is going to get. Sometimes, I will be in a lot of pain but decide to go ahead with plans, dosing myself up and keeping myself hydrated of course, and in a couple of hours the medication has helped and I feel well able to manage. Other times, I'll do that exact same thing and find that nothing helps and I feel worse and now I'm nowhere near my bed. It's a really unpleasant roulette.

I've worked it out by creating boundaries around the risk. I won't do anything that would involve danger to me or someone else if I end up feeling worse: I don't drive anywhere unless I'm confident my migraine is under control. I always take my medications and a bottle of water with me. And then, if the worst happens, I remind myself I am not in any danger and I will survive it, even if it feels absolutely horrible.

It helps that the roulette falls in my favour more often that not. The times I've gone ahead and done something anyway, and then felt either better or the same, do outweigh the times I've ended up feeling worse. I remind myself that my average pain score was for a long time a 7, and I can get myself through that. I'm kind of an expert. I think this makes me feel less afraid of the pain.

I also try to think of it in terms of what will reduce my stress. Doing anything when you have a really bad migraine will amp up your cortisol and ultimately be unhelpful in terms of delaying recovery. However, it can be *more* stressful to miss the thing you were desperate not to miss. So sometimes taking the cortisol hit from pushing yourself to do something is better than the cortisol hit from missing out/letting the side down.

Just as long as you're not *always* choosing to push through things and never rest – that would definitely be taking the "do it anyway" mentality too far. But doing it anyway under certain circumstances definitely works for me.

Dark glasses and eye shades

Dark glasses are the migraine sufferer's best friend. Even in the middle of December, you might find you need them. I never leave home without dark glasses, even on the greyest, foggiest day. That's partly because I live in the UK, where the weather changes constantly and you can find yourself going from autumnal to midsummer conditions in the course of a couple of hours, but partly because even in average brightness, dark glasses can be a great help.

Don't worry about looking pretentious. You're either coping with or preventing a migraine, which makes you pretty awesome. Other migraine sufferers will spot you, and they will be giving you sympathetic looks. You just can't see them, because they're also behind their dark glasses.

Eye shades – those comfy masks people wear on planes to try to get some sleep in the least sleep conducive environment known to humans – are also your friend, and not just when travelling. Ideally you have extremely heavy and light blocking bedroom curtains but, if you don't, a decent eye mask is much cheaper than buying some. The best ones have a soft cushiony feel around the eyes and an adjustable head strap. Also, somewhat obviously, a good quality black one will cut out more light than any other.

You can also take it with you whenever you're away from home, so no need to worry about hotel rooms or guest rooms with flimsy curtains that don't do the job and have been chosen by carefree people who are untouched by migraines.

You might also find that yellow tinted glasses help you with driving, especially at night. One of my triggers is headlights on cars coming towards me at night. They absolutely blind me and it feels like the light is cutting into my eye. I know that sounds dramatic but a car coming towards me with full beams on has immediately set off a migraine several times in the past. The yellow tinted glasses allow you to see perfectly but filter out some of the brightness of the headlights.

Ear plugs and noise cancelling headphones

While you're shopping for eye masks, get yourself some ear plugs. My ears must be a weird shape because I can't wear in-ear headphones without discomfort/them falling out, so I prefer those soft squishy earplugs that you buy in boxes of 50 and dispose of after a few uses. They fill my weird old ears and block out a lot (not everything, but they do help).

I will wear these in all kinds of situations: when I can't sleep because the migraine is bad, they dampen noise; when I am trying to sleep either because the pain is moderate or I'm recovering from a migraine, they cut down the likelihood of being disturbed; and during the day, if I choose to be up and about with a migraine and my environment is not quiet.

Noise cancelling headphones are also great. During the day, you might find not only do they cut out noise if you're trying to carry on while migraining, but that they also act as a signal to others not to ask you unnecessary questions. If you can sleep with noise cancelling headphones on (maybe you've got normal ears, I don't know) then I'm sure they're brilliant for that as well.

Music

I love my music but I usually don't want to listen to anything when I've got a migraine. However, I have discovered a thing on YouTube called Music for Migraines[xxxii] which actually isn't bad. Usually I'm totally sceptical about these things, and ready to scorn the claim that some plinky plonky music could possibly make any difference to anything as complicated as a migraine.

However, I stumbled across some tracks using delta binaural beats and found these did seem to help me feel better if I listened to them through headphones while lying in the dark. The science behind this is that since binaural beats give the right and left ear sounds at slightly different frequencies, the brain is tricked into changing its activity[xxxiii]. In the case of delta binaural beats, the brain is encouraged to prepare for sleep. I certainly felt that it helped to slow my racing thoughts and relax in spite of pain.

It's one of those things that might be a 5-10% solution for you – it might make things a small but significant bit better.

Ice packs

Something else you might consider keeping to hand is ice packs. If migraines are caused or made worse by blood vessels dilating, a bit of cold therapy can have the effect of temporarily constricting a small area. It won't cure your migraine or even temporarily erase it, but you can expect it to give you a little bit of relief.

An ice pack held to whichever side of the head your migraine is on, especially over the eyebrow, can give you that little bit of vasoconstriction and/or numb the pain slightly. Keep a bunch in your freezer for whenever you need them.

You can also buy instant ice packs that you carry around and activate when you need them. They are single use sachets that go cold as soon as you squeeze and shake them, and stay cold for about 15 minutes – first aiders often carry them, but they're just as good for migraines.

You can even buy such things made into hats. I've never tried this but it is tempting.

Thought games for the anxiety

I've made up a number of thought games to play for when my mind is racing, as it tends to do as the pain ramps up. Sometimes it's racing because of the pain and I'm panicking about how it will cope if it gets any worse, and sometimes it's racing because of all the things I should be doing/need to catch up on/will have to make alternative plans for because I can't do them right now.

Needless to say, none of these speedy trains of thought helps with migraine pain at all. So I've found some things that are much gentler to let my thoughts meander around.

I like stories a lot, so I let myself cook up stories in my head. These are not complex thrillers with clever turns, layered characters and a plot twist you'll never see coming. They are quite childish and silly and simple, because that is what you need when you have a migraine.

I start with three things: a noun, a verb and an adjective. Rabbit jumping purple. Rainbow snoring gigantic. Parsnip driving beautiful. Then I try to make a scene or story out of my random words. Maybe I invent a purple rabbit who is jumping through fields. Oh, she's purple because they are beetroot fields and she's got carried away. Perhaps there is a giant rainbow snoring because there hasn't been any rain or sun in a while – there could be a whole story around who wakes it up, and how. Or maybe the snores are gigantic, and sound like thunder, and the moon and the sun and the clouds have to club together and send the rainbow to a sleep clinic. Oh, there goes a car made out of parsnips, it's driving beautifully...OK, some of these may have more mileage (sorry) than others, but you get the idea.

There is something about playing with your thoughts and imagination that puts us on a different track. It's hard to feel anxious when you're imagining a purple rabbit scrubbing off beetroot stains in a bubble bath. Or at least it's hard to feel as anxious as you did a moment ago when you were instead thinking about walking the dog, taking the kids swimming, picking up more bread and milk, rearranging your work day, figuring out whether today is a triptan day or not...

There is also my alphabet game, decorating the empty house and time travelling (see **Sleep**). But any gentle thought train will do. Anything that feels playful and gentle.

You might even come up with an amazing children's book. Migraine brains are not good at remembering things or thinking logically, but they might just invent a parsnip driving a beautiful gang of crime fighting vegetables around town.

Be prepared with your migraine first aid kit

You'll have gathered by now that my handbag is quite a large one. Every time I leave the house, it needs to contain:
- Paracetamol and ibuprofen
- An OTC codeine containing painkiller
- Triptans
- A bottle of water
- Dark glasses
- Ear plugs
- A portable ice pack
- As well as all the other completely necessary items I carry around, like my wallet, phone, keys, tissues, hand sanitiser, hand cream, lip balm, sanitary towels, umbrella, snack, pens, current book etc

However, a slightly strained shoulder is a small price to pay for knowing I always have stuff on hand for a migraine attack. It's saved me a number of times, just having the right medication to hand while out, or having my dark glasses or earplugs in reach.

If you can stretch to it, have enough of all these things that you never have to take them out of your handbag, i.e. you've got more painkillers/another pair of dark glasses in the house. That way you don't have to remember each time to pack your kit: it's already there. It will help enormously when you are mid migraine and you can't think clearly. Think of it as a favour your well self can do for your future not so well self.

Think about where you need these things in your house, too. Dark glasses by the back door are useful for me, as is having a few painkillers in my bedside drawer as well as the main stash in my kitchen. I also have a few in my therapy room, in case pain comes on at work. There's another pair of dark glasses that live in the car, along with a yellow tinted pair that I just use for driving at night.

Just make things as easy and convenient for your poor migraining self as you possibly can. And never leave home without your migraine kit.

Expect a migraine

I'm not saying get all gloomy about it and take the stance that you're always going to have a migraine. But it will often show up at the least convenient times, i.e. times when you're stressed or excited or doing something different, because we know those are key migraine triggers.

Migraine *will* show up when you go on holiday. In the past ten years I have taken a dozen flights and only one of them was migraine-free. This is partly the excitement of going on holiday, partly the "let down" effect of having time off, partly a bit of anxiety about travel arrangements and wondering if I packed everything, and partly that my migraines just *are* triggered by anything out of the ordinary. I've learned to accept that this is part of travelling, which I most certainly do not want to stop doing, and to fly with my migraine kit in my hand luggage.

Migraine always shows up in the sunshine for me, too, and although we don't always take breaks in sunny places, we often do. I'm also very fair skinned so I've got two good reasons to seek the shade. It's actually pretty easy to do this around the pool or on the beach (the beach umbrella is your friend) but when you are out in the sun, a hat and dark glasses are essential. This applies whether you have a migraine starting, a full blown migraine attack or no migraine at all. Have your migraine kit handy at all times, drink *even more* water than usual, and take every excuse for a nap. You're on holiday after all!

The migraine is no respecter of your once in a lifetime trip, either. Two years ago we went to Florida and did all the parks, which was absolutely brilliant and a real one-time-only thing. One of the days I had been looking forward to the most was the one at the water park. We're all swimmers and love piling down flumes and all of that lark. But this was one place where there was very little shade – the only option was to fork out $100 for a sunbed in the shade – and I thought "I'll be OK!" Which naturally I wasn't. At the first sign of pain I took my ibuprofen and clattered down a flume or two. I didn't mess about with it – when the pain ramped up within half an hour (largely due, I'm sure, to spending that half hour in a sunny queue for a flume ride) I took my triptan. This was definitely a triptan day.

I thought a triptan and a big drink would sort it. It did not. By lunchtime I was at a 10 on the pain scale because although I'd taken a triptan I'd also been relentlessly in full sun, in a very noisy place, and you simply cannot wear sunglasses on flumes, people. (You can get dark goggles, mind you, which I would recommend).

I was in so much pain I had to remind myself to breathe. It was intense. We found some shade at a cafe so that my husband and daughter could eat lunch and I could get out of the sun for a bit. We all hoped that a lemonade would help me out – I knew it wouldn't, but it bought me some time in the shade while I hoped desperately that the triptan would do something.

My husband decided that $100 was a completely reasonable and necessary spend if I were to have any chance of bouncing back to participate in the rest of the day, so we got the world's most pricey umbrella and I collapsed on a lounger under it with a towel over my face. I threw down some codeine so I'd know I'd given everything I possibly could, and my husband and daughter left me for an hour.

Somehow, to a soundtrack of screams, laughter, a wave machine siren and a constant stream of Beach Boys hits, I slipped into a weird state on the edge of sleep where I guess gradually one of the things I'd taken (or maybe all of them) began to work. An hour later, I emerged from the towel, able to tolerate the afternoon light and drink another pint of fluids. I felt so much better. I went and did all the rides I'd missed out on, and we stayed extra late so I could catch up and squeeze the most out of the day. It was alright in the end.

But it could have gone the other way. It could so easily have been that nothing I tried worked and I was stuck under that towel for the rest of the afternoon, and we probably would have packed up and gone back to the hotel early, and everyone would have been sorry about it. Because sometimes there is nothing you can do but wait. Even on the most special of days that you've been looking forward to for a long time.

Knowing that it might happen doesn't make it any easier for you, or for anyone else. But somehow I am glad that I know to expect it. It gives me a chance to formulate a plan of what I *might* do, even if I've no guarantee that plan will work. And it gives me and my family a chance to adjust for how things might go if I am incapacitated.

There is something for me about accepting that I have migraines and that they can show up at any time, no matter how well I plan or hope for the best. I think possibly it takes the stress down a tiny notch. By the time the migraine arrives, at the worst juncture it could, I am not also internally screaming it down for having the audacity to show up. I am not pleased it's here, either, far from it – but there is a degree of neutrality that is probably helpful for trying to stay calm and saving my energy for managing pain.

Ways I've managed (bad)

Making no concessions for myself

There have been times when I've decided to carry on as though I didn't have a migraine. Sometimes doing things in spite of a migraine can be the best thing I can do, but what I've been very bad at doing sometimes is carrying on as normal *without making any concessions for myself whatsoever*.

What I mean by this is that I haven't told anyone I have a migraine, nor have I done anything different to help myself.

Something that's easy peasy when I'm well, like making dinner for example, can be a bit of a challenge when I have a migraine.

Once, making no concessions for myself whatsoever, I cracked on with making a lovely dinner that involved a stew and homemade bread. This is what doing it with no concessions looked like:
- I worked through the steps of the recipe without taking any breaks, and maybe even attempted to do that devil's work, multitasking.
- I cut my finger while prepping the veg because my hand-eye coordination is terrible when I have a migraine.
- When trying to brown the meat, I burned it, because my brain couldn't keep track of when it needed to be turned.
- I burned myself putting the heavy stew pot into the oven because gross motor movements don't always work out so well with migraine either.
- I made my pain worse kneading dough because that's actually quite hard physical work and all bakers are pretty buff.
- The bread wasn't ready at the same time as the stew because coordinating timings, even simple ones, is just tough with a migraine.
- I left out a couple of the herbs because I just didn't read the recipe right. Happens to us all but more likely at migraine time.
- I was grumpy as well as in pain by the time it was ready, which didn't make the prospect of trying to eat something any easier, nor did it make me a nicer member of the family to sit down with.

And here's what doing it whilst making concessions for myself looks like:
- I tell my family that I have a migraine. I'm going to make dinner like I planned, as I think I can manage most of it, but I put them on standby to assist me if I need it.

- I realise I do need assistance and I ask someone else to do the sharp knife stuff while I give browning the meat my full attention.
- Even with full attention, we're talking full *migraine* attention, so I set a (quiet) timer to go off when I need to do something important – one less thing to attempt to hold in my poor aching brain.
- I work slower, and stop to glug water and nibble on the veggies before they go in the pot.
- I might assemble everything I need for the entire recipe on the counter before I start, so I am less likely to forget something. Or get someone else to do this. And if herbs get left out, forgive yourself, they're only herbs.
- Definitely get someone else to put the heavy casserole in the oven. If you don't burn yourself, you'll probably spill the whole lot on the floor, and that's just heartbreaking (although not for the dog).
- Naff off to the shop for the bread (or send someone if the shop is a drive away). Making bread is for well people. And buff bakers.
- If timings matter, talk them out loud to someone else, who can check your maths with a clear head.
- Sit down feeling like you've achieved something, that you didn't have to do it all by yourself, and that you just might be able to eat some of it.

Never cancelling work

Look, don't take this the wrong way, but...you're not that important. People will cope without you!

I say this as a person who helps people with their mental health, and sometimes people come into my office having some pretty dire problems with their mental health. It can feel very compelling to be there at all costs. When your clients are dealing with trauma, grief, abuse, addictions, eating disorders, family rifts, illness, prejudice, loss and anxiety, it's easy to feel "Well, it's just a migraine."

No matter what our job, we all have ways in which we feel sure we are indispensable, that things will go horribly wrong if we're not there, and that we'll be letting people down horribly if we don't show up.

And my clients have been sorry, annoyed or angry sometimes when I haven't been able to be with them. But they've also managed. They've had a chance to work out how to manage without their session that week. When we come back together, I ask them about how that was and encourage them to tell me about it honestly. Sometimes it transpires that they were furious with me and we get to talking about what that reminded them of. Other times they found some other way of coping, maybe not one we want to continue working on, or maybe an excellent one that hadn't occurred to them before. They're always alright though. Of course they are. I'm not *that* important.

All therapists who take their job seriously have a supervisor, a more experienced therapist than themselves who they meet with once a month and whose job it is to help them work through any sticking points and check on their general wellbeing. Because working as a therapist involves bringing so much of what makes you *you* to work, the general mental and physical health of the therapist tends to correlate to how well they're about to work, so paying attention to wellbeing is important.

My supervisor is well aware that I am not very good at cancelling work, so she turned the tables on me. When she was ill, and had to cancel two sessions in a fairly short space of time, she asked me how I had felt about it.

I can be honest with her but truly, I had thought about it so little that I had to take a moment to check what I really did feel about it.

See? It was so OK with me that she cancelled due to illness that I had hardly needed to think about it.

And, when I did think about it, I realised I was glad she'd trusted me enough to cancel. I hated the thought of her trying to make a session work while she didn't feel well enough to be there. Partly, she knew I'd be alright. And partly, I knew I'd be alright. I can't tell other colleagues about my clients because of confidentiality, but if I'd needed to talk over anything personal to do with my own wellbeing, I had other options for that. She knew I'd exercise my judgement and put things in place for myself.

That was quite confidence inspiring, really: I respect my supervisor a great deal and think she's incredibly wise. Therefore I believed she was right and I liked that she had that trust in me. I hope my clients might feel this to some degree when I cancel on them.

Of course, I am talking about the occasional cancellation, and not being unable to work for weeks or months at a time. You might find yourself in a different situation, where you really can't work for a spell. Maybe your job doesn't involve sitting quietly in a room with just one other person. Maybe you are dealing with migraines while your job involves noisy machinery, or climbing ladders or teaching five year olds.

I can't tell you what to do, and I'm not even going to pretend that there are any easy or right answers. All I can say is, after ten years of working whilst migraining, I look back and think that I could definitely have taken more time off. I'm not sorry for the times I made it, and I don't regret making the stretch to be there. But if I hadn't made it, it probably would have been OK.

Exercise

Exercise is a great thing for all sorts of reasons, none of which I'm going to go into here. It can even be something that doesn't make a migraine worse, if you keep to very gentle things like a walk or a bit of yoga or stretching.

In my experience, any other kind of exercise during a migraine is to be avoided.

I have tried to "do it anyway" by going for a run (what was I thinking? My head felt like it was going to split in half every time my foot hit the pavement), going for a swim (within one length, the pain in my head lit up like a Christmas tree and I went from a 3 to an 8) and, once, doing a cartwheel (I puked. It was not pretty).

Also, any vigorous exercise is a reliable trigger for me. I could have no migraine pain at all and feel completely well, but one exercise class later my head will be throbbing and on fire.

Exercises that don't trigger me include walking, gentle cycling, gentle swimming and yoga. Happily, these are all exercises I like. I did used to run but I always hated it so when I was forced to give up because of migraines I was secretly delighted.

Adriene Mishler runs a free yoga channel on YouTube[xxxiv] full of totally accessible home yoga, which I would recommend to anyone. Also, Joe Wicks has made some workouts specifically for perimenopausal women[xxxv] which use stretching and weights and feel as though they're pitched just right.

Maybe you're one of those people who gets endorphin rushes when you exercise, and no migraine at all. In which case, exercise might be far more helpful than harmful to you in managing things. I always felt rather cheated that I never felt endorphins (I really deserved them for running) but maybe it has to do with not enjoying sport, despite coming from a sporty family. I am the odd one out who likes nothing better than reading a book, and I'm sure book endorphins are a thing.

Overt violence

Migraine pain has sometimes been so relentless and difficult to cope with that I have occasionally punched myself as hard as I can in the head.

Luckily I am a bit of a wimp and haven't done myself much harm.

I know that this will sound a bit unhinged to you, especially if you've never had a migraine, or any kind of pain that takes over for days at a time. But clients have talked to me about this exact same thing. I've heard stories of people slamming their head against a wall or giving themselves a good whack with a saucepan. It's quite a natural consequence of being driven to despair by pain.

Obviously I wouldn't recommend it. Apart from anything else, the thinking behind it is faulty. I know I thought I could replace one pain (the migraine) with another (being punched). But it simply doesn't work like that. If you don't believe me, next time you have a migraine, get an ice cube out of the freezer and try holding it in your hand until it melts. Chances are, you won't be able to hold it for that long, because it hurts a lot. Did it get rid of your migraine though? No, I thought not. And if it did distract you from the pain for a minute or two, then at least you've only injured an ice cube, and not your head.

Dr Google

If you Google "Can my migraine kill me?" or "Could my migraine be a brain tumour?" the answer will be yes. I know you will Google this stuff anyway because I did and still do.

Stupid things people say about migraine

People are lovely really, and they just want to help fix things. Therefore, a lot of the stupid things people have said to me about migraine have begun with the words *Have you tried...?* Here are some things that well meaning people have asked me.
"Have you tried deep breaths?"
Sure. I'm trying them right now, as I restrain myself from slapping you.
"Have you tried a sugar free diet?"
I mean, when the cure is worse than the migraine, it's just not worth it, is it? To dodge this kind of comment, throw a handful of M&Ms at the well-meaning rice-cake eater and run for your life. You can run quite slowly because they won't have the energy to run after you.
"Have you tried cannabis?"
Illegal solutions are a no-no for me, personally. I'm not judging people who use them and, if they work for you, I can see why you'd go there. But, for a variety of reasons, I'm not breaking the law. Also, I've done enough work with addicts to know that cannabis is not the soft drug or easy ride that it seems to be pitched as, either. The withdrawal is hell. And, being in perimenopause, I'm already dealing with a hefty helping of brain fog. I can probably do without cannabis adding to that.
"Have you tried praying?"
I am not here to knock anyone's religious belief. If you believe in something, I can absolutely see how it will comfort you in the midst of a migraine to be in commune with that something, to perhaps feel the presence of something to help you bear the suffering. But I do not think praying is going to take anyone's migraine away.
"Have you tried crystals?"
Apparently you can pop them on your windowsill, and/or carry them in your pockets. Possibly if I was nine years old, this would

appeal. But I doubt even a nine year old would imagine that owning a crystal would prevent a migraine.

"Have you tried wearing a magnetic bracelet?"
See above.

"Have you tried acupuncture?"
Much as I enjoy an alternative remedy or two, I don't think acupuncture (or homeopathy or Reiki) has a place in treating something as painful as migraine. If something's a little off, and realigning your energy or rubbing on a bit of peppermint tincture helps, then great. But if you have a big, booming migraine, it's going to be useless.

Unless, perhaps, you really believe in it. Clearly, I am a sceptic. However, plenty of research suggests that acupuncture for chronic pain is just marginally better than a placebo when it comes to reducing the frequency of migraines[xxxvi].

Placebos, it's well known, can be powerful – they certainly benefit us more than doing nothing. This is largely because if we expect something to happen, we look for confirmation that it is happening, and are more likely to actively notice that we have less pain or fewer attacks. I think this might be why acupuncture, or any other alternative medicine, works well for some people. If you think acupuncture will help, then it just might do. If you're a sceptic, it almost certainly won't help at all.

"Have you tried relaxing?"
You know, I have. It's just that it's really impossible with a booming head, a sicky tummy and a spinning room. Tell me more about spa days, though. That does sound pretty good for when I'm well again.

Other unhelpful things people have said to me
"You don't look like you have a migraine."
People with migraines don't always appear on the horizon wearing dark glasses and clutching an ice pack to their heads. Some of the time they are just trying to get through their day at

work while hoping the triptan or drug of choice they took earlier will hurry up and provide them some relief.

During my worst migraines, I have felt like there *should* be some visible sign that my head feels like it's about to burst. There's some very relatable migraine art out there that depicts fault lines running across foreheads and through temples, with dramatic cracks and splits. But the truth is, sometimes the eye on the affected side waters, and that's about the extent of the visual clues.

This applies to a whole host of things, both physical and not, but you really can't tell by looking at someone what they're going through on the inside. If they say they have a migraine, even if they currently seem to be nailing it, believe them.

"Is it your ponytail?"
People have given themselves headaches from putting their hair up too tightly. That's real. But no, wearing a ponytail does not cause a migraine. If it did, I would just wear my hair loose every day and be migraine free.

People with migraines are in pain and might be cognitively impaired during attacks, but we're not stupid. If it was down to something as simple as that, we'd all be skipping down sunlit beaches without eye protection whilst listening to loud music.

Hope for the future

As I write this in 2024, a new family of migraine prevention drugs called gepants have just been approved by NICE for use in the UK. They are the first preventative drug designed specifically for migraine[xxxvii].

Prior to this, the three main migraine prevention options are Amitriptyline (originally designed for anxiety and depression), beta blockers (which primarily treat heart conditions) and Topiramate (for epilepsy). While these preventatives can often be of real help to migraine sufferers, it is surely even better to finally have something specifically designed for the 15% of the population affected by migraine.

The newest gepant, called Atogepant, works by blocking the nerve receptors that make us feel pain during migraine attacks, and they specifically target receptors called Calcitonin Gene-Related Peptide (CGRP). It has been proven to prevent migraine attack severity and frequency, with fewer side effects that some of the preventative treatments we might have tried before[xxxviii].

It is only available on prescription so, if you want to try it for your migraines, your first step is to make an appointment with your GP. You will need to discuss your migraine history and any previous treatments so that your doctor can determine whether Atogepant might be suitable for you.

If you're worried about pronouncing it correctly, it is pronounced "Gee, pants!" and not "geh-pants", and so Atogepant is "A-toe-gee-pant" although I have heard it said more along the lines of "A toga pant" as well. Your GP will know what you mean.

What I have learned from perimenopausal migraines

I'm not one for believing that everything happens for a reason, nor that suffering makes us stronger. Therefore I feel quite wary writing about what I might have gained from migraines, because it suggests that all migraineurs should just shutup and accept that this is all for the best somehow. I hope you've gathered from the rest of this book that I am really way more sympathetic than that when it comes to migraines.

However, there is something I've noticed now that I'm getting better that I had never experienced before, and it offered me a little glimpse into what I might have learned from chronic pain.

The first time my migraine diary recorded two weeks without a migraine I was ecstatic, hopeful and a bit on edge, to be honest. I was glad to have had the pain-free respite, obviously, and it meant that physically I felt pretty good. But I also knew it meant that the next attack was probably just around the corner as I just hadn't gone a fortnight without a migraine in such a long time.

I was right, of course. The next migraine popped up the very next day. But, as I got used to the occasional two week migraine free stretch, and then it began to happen with some frequency, a new feeling crept in – one that's much harder to admit to.

Sometimes...I missed my migraines.

That's wild, isn't it? These horrible things that had caused me so much pain, made me skip nice things, seen me struggle through things that had to get done, not being able to sleep...I'd have to be an absolute buffoon to miss any of that.

Of course, I wasn't missing the pain or the inconvenience. I had come to rely on migraines as a time to slow down. I mean, I *had* to slow down when in that much pain. And, because I never knew when the next attack was coming, I was treating the time inbetween as the time to catch up on all that I'd missed as well as trying to get ahead so I minimised the disruption from the next migraine. I ended up never slowing down when I was well.

I suppose I was always a naturally quite fast-paced person. My thoughts jog along quite quickly, I like it when I can get things done rapidly and I quite enjoy having a fair bit to do. Counselling taught me that sometimes this is about avoiding quiet reflection time because it might bring things forward that I don't want to look at, but then counselling also taught me that when I did slow down and reflect I could handle things. So I always had the option to slow down but...I wouldn't often choose to. I think that is just how I am built.

However, if running too fast too often was part of what triggered a migraine, and if I was secretly missing those times when migraines forced me to slow down, well then maybe slowing down was something I needed to work on. It might not be my natural set point, but we can all stretch to try different things and learn other ways. I started to let myself slow down when there was no migraine. Not even a slight gnawing at my temple.

This looked very small at first. For example I will often, when waiting for the kettle to boil for my (decaf) brew, use the time to empty the dishwasher. I'm like "I bet I can get the whole lot put away before this kettle boils" and then it becomes a daft little challenge. I tear around stacking plates and stashing cutlery and yes, I nearly always beat the kettle. So I stopped doing that. My kitchen window is right there and it looks out onto the back garden, where there are nearly always cats, squirrels or birds providing free entertainment. The first time I did this, I promise you, I saw a squirrel nick a pear from nextdoor's tree, hang upside down from one of our trees, and tuck into its purloined bounty. I'm sure the dishwasher got emptied some other time.

When I have a migraine, I literally can't do two things at once. I can barely do the one thing I'm attempting to do. So I stopped doing more than one thing at once at other times. Just because I can text my friend whilst making dinner, doesn't mean I should. Actually it feels a lot better to sit down and text her when I'm giving the message my full attention and properly reading what she sent me. Maybe it means I text less often, but that's OK. And maybe the dinner gets burned less often, too.

I tried (I still try) to make this work for bigger things. When my daughter or my husband are talking to me, I want to slow down by stopping what I'm doing and giving them my full attention. Often they'll say a lot more if I'm doing that. I'll take it in better and probably respond in a more attuned way. (The exception to this is when a teenager is trying to talk about something you sense makes them feel awkward: then it really helps them out if they think you're actually looking at the laundry you're folding).

And I don't have to catch up on all the things I missed when I was too sick to participate. It shouldn't work like that. I try to work out what it is essential to catch up on, and what can be left, given to someone else or done in a less onerous way.

Ultimately I think that's being kind to myself. Even if it had no impact on how many migraines I have, it was worth doing for that reason alone.

So migraine has taught me that slowing down is necessary. It's even nice. That's what I was missing when I thought I was missing have so many migraines. So, as long as I remind myself to slow down on a regular basis, life feels better.

For the same reason, on days when medication makes me feel so much better – even totally better – I try not to behave as though I can do everything. I am grateful that medication frequently allows me to carry on with work and family life when I otherwise wouldn't have been able to, but I try not to take liberties by packing out my schedule and thinking "Well, the painkillers/triptans will get me through." If perimenopausal migraine is trying to tell me that my body is going through a huge change, then I guess it makes sense to allow a bit of space for that change to happen. It's hard to manage a big change when your schedule is bursting and you're filling your every waking moment with stuff you need to do.

I have read accounts of women taking time out, or a "menopause gap year" if you will, and I don't feel so sure about that. Even if I had the kind of job and the kind of money to do that, I doubt I'd choose it. For me, staying connected to family and work life and friends is incredibly important, even if I can't do it as much or in all the ways I'd like.

I know some people sail through perimenopause without much trouble and, if you are one of the people who doesn't, either because you have crippling migraines or one of the host of other awful symptoms this time of life can gift you, it can feel very unfair. But it's really just that your body is more sensitive to hormonal changes. I have a feeling that I'm built in a way that means I will always feel the rollercoaster of hormonal tomfoolery. I may be able to smooth the ride somewhat by trying to slow down and look after myself, but I can't cut out the impact completely. Part of my job here is to accept this is my thing and talk myself up to manage it.

Also, let's come back to the TEN YEARS thing that I mentioned at the start of this book. If perimenopausal symptoms last about a decade, then we are coming out the other side of this. Sometime after we've gone through menopause, and no longer have periods to deal with (a boon in and of itself) we will very likely also no longer have all these other symptoms caused by our punk rock hormones. Post menopausal women tell me this is like having a new lease of life. They are finally free of the difficulties being sensitive to hormonal changes have caused them, leaving so much more time for them to get on with whatever else takes their fancy.

That sounds brilliant to me. If we're lucky, we might expect to live another three decades post menopause, which is a lovely long stretch of time to fill with whatever it is people do when they don't have perimenopausal migraines.

Acknowledgements

Thanks enormously to my dear friend and early reader, Marie. Your kind words push me on in all the best ways.

Thanks also to my fellow writer and counselling colleague, Laura, who was so generous as to share her own writing journey with me and give me feedback on my own drafts. I couldn't have wished for a better mentor! (Check out her wonderful books about parenting teens here: http://www.laurathomascounselling.co.uk/parenting-teens/)

Always thankful for Tricia, my supervisor and long-time collaborator – there's no problem too thorny for her, she unfailingly makes things clearer. Every therapist needs a Tricia.

Thanks to Sarah, for always listening, even when she's heard it all before and there are no answers. I love our catch up dinners so much!

Thanks to Dr Foo, the GP who really listened and understood, always wanting to make things better.

I'm indebted to Ann-Marie, for that conversation in the garden at the family reunion. You told me to write, and I have!

Debt of gratitude to my friend and fellow writer Steve who offered much support and guided me through my more stupid technical questions.

Thanks also to my other friends who have been willing to talk perimeno over all manner of non-caffeinated soft drinks: Vic, Jo, Debs, Ali, Belle, Frances and Nat.

Grateful to all my clients, who teach me so many things every day. I feel very fortunate to be able to do this job.

Biggest thanks always to Ian and Kate, whose love and support has been unfailing. I really lucked out with you both. Boop!

About the author

I am a therapist practising in Cambridge UK, writing books in my spare time. I have a decade of experience as a therapist, but have been writing books since I was in primary school. Early "publications" (one handwritten copy, passed around the playground) included such illustrious titles as *The Poo Squirters*. Maybe my writing has become slightly more sophisticated since then: you be the judge of that.

I live in the beautiful city of Cambridge with my husband, our daughter and two very cute cats. When I am not working or writing, you will find me with my head in a book.

You can find me at www.kirsty-campbell.com

References

[i] World Health Organisation https://www.who.int/news-room/fact-sheets/detail/headache-disorders

[ii] British Menopause Association https://thebms.org.uk/wp-content/uploads/2022/12/06-BMS-TfC-Migraine-and-HRT-NOV2022-A.pdf

[iii] Wattieze et al, Wattiez AS, Sowers LP, Russo AF. Calcitonin gene-related peptide (CGRP): role in migraine pathophysiology and therapeutic targeting. Expert Opin Ther Targets. 2020 Feb;24(2):91-100. doi: 10.1080/14728222.2020.1724285. Epub 2020 Feb 13. PMID: 32003253; PMCID: PMC7050542.

[iv] The Migraine Trust https://migrainetrust.org/understand-migraine/genetics-and-migraine/

[v] The Cleveland Clinic https://my.clevelandclinic.org/health/diseases/5005-migraine-headaches

[vi] Society for Womens Health Research https://swhr.org/menopause-perimenopause-and-migraine/

[vii] Elinor Cleghorn, *Unwell Women*

[viii] Womens Health Concern https://www.womens-health-concern.org/wp-content/uploads/2023/11/18-WHC-FACTSHEET-Migraine-and-HRT-NOV2023-B.pdf

[ix] National Migraine Centre https://www.nationalmigrainecentre.org.uk/understanding-migraine/factsheets-and-resources/migraine-menopause-and-hrt/

[x] The Cleveland Clinic https://my.clevelandclinic.org/health/treatments/24998-triptans

[xi] Malhotra R. Understanding migraine: Potential role of neurogenic inflammation. Ann Indian Acad Neurol. 2016 Apr-Jun;19(2):175-82. doi: 10.4103/0972-2327.182302. PMID: 27293326; PMCID: PMC4888678.

[xii] Woldeamanuel YW, Sanjanwala BM, Cowan RP. Endogenous glucocorticoids may serve as biomarkers for migraine chronification. Ther Adv Chronic Dis. 2020 Jul 21;11:2040622320939793. doi: 10.1177/2040622320939793. PMID: 32973989; PMCID: PMC7495027.

[xiii] Womens Health Concern https://www.womens-health-concern.org/wp-content/uploads/2023/11/18-WHC-FACTSHEET-Migraine-and-HRT-NOV2023-B.pdf

xiv The Menopause Charity https://www.themenopausecharity.org/2021/10/21/what-is-hormone-replacement-therapy-hrt/

xv Ibid

xvi NHS UK https://www.nhs.uk/medicines/hormone-replacement-therapy-hrt/benefits-and-risks-of-hormone-replacement-therapy-hrt/

xvii NHS UK https://www.nhs.uk/conditions/menopause/treatment/

xviii University of Oxford https://www.psych.ox.ac.uk/news/triptans-found-to-be-the-most-effective-drug-for-acute-migraine-sufferers

xix The Migraine Trust https://migrainetrust.org/live-with-migraine/healthcare/treatments/acute-medicines/

xx House of Commons Library https://commonslibrary.parliament.uk/research-briefings/cdp-2024-0060/

xxi Headache Log, Created and developed by AR Productions (I found it on the Google Play app)

xxii Addicott MA, Yang LL, Peiffer AM, Burnett LR, Burdette JH, Chen MY, Hayasaka S, Kraft RA, Maldjian JA, Laurienti PJ. The effect of daily caffeine use on cerebral blood flow: How much caffeine can we tolerate? Hum Brain Mapp. 2009 Oct;30(10):3102-14. doi: 10.1002/hbm.20732. PMID: 19219847; PMCID: PMC2748160.

xxiii Healthline https://www.healthline.com/health/throbbing-headache

xxiv Rehabs UK https://rehabsuk.com/blog/how-alcohol-is-linked-to-headaches-and-migraines/

xxv American Migraine Foundation https://americanmigrainefoundation.org/resource-library/migraine-let-down-headache/

xxvi Herrera AY, Nielsen SE, Mather M. Stress-induced increases in progesterone and cortisol in naturally cycling women. Neurobiol Stress. 2016 Feb 11;3:96-104. doi: 10.1016/j.ynstr.2016.02.006. PMID: 27981182; PMCID: PMC5146195.

xxvii Rape Crisis UK https://rapecrisis.org.uk/get-informed/statistics-sexual-violence/

xxviii Daniunaite I, Cloitre M, Karatzias T, Shevlin M, Thoresen S, Zelviene P, Kazlauskas E. PTSD and complex PTSD in adolescence: discriminating factors in a population-based cross-sectional study. Eur J Psychotraumatol. 2021 Mar 30;12(1):1890937. doi: 10.1080/20008198.2021.1890937. PMID: 33968323; PMCID: PMC8075084.

xxix Severn Clinics https://severnclinics.co.nz/trauma-and-the-limbic-system/

xxx   Cleveland Clinic https://my.clevelandclinic.org/health/diseases/24881-cptsd-complex-ptsd

xxxi   Hannibal KE, Bishop MD. Chronic stress, cortisol dysfunction, and pain: a psychoneuroendocrine rationale for stress management in pain rehabilitation. Phys Ther. 2014 Dec;94(12):1816-25. doi: 10.2522/ptj.20130597. Epub 2014 Jul 17. PMID: 25035267; PMCID: PMC4263906.

xxxii   https://www.youtube.com/watch?v=5jmrIggwCXc&t=1108s

xxxiii   The Migraine Relief Center https://blog.themigrainereliefcenter.com/binaural-beats-and-migraines-what-you-need-to-know

xxxiv   https://www.youtube.com/@yogawithadriene

xxxv   https://www.youtube.com/@TheBodyCoachTV

xxxvi   Giannini G, Favoni V, Merli E, Nicodemo M, Torelli P, Matrà A, Giovanardi CM, Cortelli P, Pierangeli G, Cevoli S. A Randomized Clinical Trial on Acupuncture Versus Best Medical Therapy in Episodic Migraine Prophylaxis: The ACUMIGRAN Study. Front Neurol. 2021 Jan 15;11:570335. doi: 10.3389/fneur.2020.570335. PMID: 33519664; PMCID: PMC7843562.

xxxvii   The Migraine Trust https://migrainetrust.org/news/nice-announces-approval-of-atogepant-for-preventive-use-on-the-nhs-in-england/

xxxviii   The Migraine Trust https://migrainetrust.org/news/gepants-for-migraine-what-are-they-and-who-might-they-be-suitable-for/

Printed in Great Britain
by Amazon